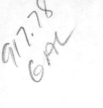

D0631005

Walking St. Louis

Judith Galas and Cindy West

AVA Endorsed by the American Volkssport Association

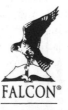

FALCON®

GUILFORD, CONNECTICUT
HELENA, MONTANA

AN IMPRINT OF THE GLOBE PEQUOT PRESS

⁄FALCONGUIDE®

ISBN 1-56044-600-5

Library of Congress Cataloging-in-Publication Data is available.

Printed in Canada
First Edition/Second Printing

CAUTION
The Globe Pequot Press assumes no liability for accidents happening to or injuries sustained by readers who engage in the activities described in this book.

To Jewell and Diane

Contents

the walks

Acknowledgments

Many people made this book possible.

Without the city walks sponsored by the St. Louis-Stuttgart Sister City Volkswalking Club, we would never have discovered St. Louis's sidewalk charm. We also thank Judy Eyerly and Dana Pahrm for being our first tour guides.

This book was enhanced considerably through the help and personal attention of the following people or offices:

— Chris Koin and Charles Dennis at the Lynch Street Bistro for sharing their enthusiasm for the Soulard area and its magic;

— Delle Willett and the Missouri Botanical Garden for gracious permission to use the garden's map;

— Donna Andrews at the St. Louis Convention and Visitors Commission for tracking down great pictures, and the commission for the wealth of information;

— Tina, the friendly information clerk at the Metro Ride store who explained the bus system and helped us find the schedules we needed;

— volkswalkers Betty Hoffman, whose great downtown and Central West End walks inspired us, and Clare Fulvio, for her historical tidbits on the Central West End;

— Elaine Pittaluga at Washington University for a photo;

— Tom Layloff for tips on places to visit;

— Bellefontaine Superintendent Mike Tiemann for his help with the cemetery walk and use of the map, and Manual Garcia for sharing his enthusiasm;

— Dale Johnson of Calvary Cemetery for help in locating graves and for use of the map;

— museum educator Jack Grothe, at Jefferson Barracks Historic Site, for sharing information;

— the helpful folks at the Greater St. Charles Convention and Visitors Bureau;

— Jo Kathman, public relations director at Our Lady of the Snows Shrine, for information and use of the map;

— and immense thanks to proofreaders and volkswalkers Andy and Linda Lucas, Dave and Edna Lanahan, Roland Klein, Sue Webb, and Vic and Fran Shaff. Your attention to detail kept us accurate.

Foreword

For almost twenty years, Falcon has guided millions of people to America's wild outside, showing them where to paddle, hike, bike, bird, fish, climb, and drive. With this walking series, we at Falcon ask you to try something just as adventurous. We invite you to experience this country from its sidewalks, not its back roads, and to stroll through some of America's most interesting cities.

In their haste to get where they are going, travelers often bypass this country's cities, and in the process, they miss the historic and scenic treasures hidden among the bricks. Many people seek spectacular scenery and beautiful settings on top of the mountains, along the rivers, and in the woods. While nothing can replace the serenity and inspiration of America's natural wonders, we should not overlook the beauty of the urban landscape.

The steel and glass of municipal mountains reflect the sunlight and make people feel small in the shadows. Birds sing in city parks, water burbles in the fountains, and along the sidewalks walkers can still see abundant wildlife—their fellow human beings.

Falcon's many outdoor guidebooks have encouraged people not only to explore and enjoy America's natural beauty but to preserve and protect it. Our cities also are meant to be enjoyed and explored, and their irreplaceable treasures need care and protection.

When travelers and walkers want to explore something that is inspirational and beautiful, we hope they will lace up their walking shoes and point their feet toward one of this country's many cities.

For there, along the walkways, they are sure to discover the excitement, history, beauty, and charm of urban America.

—*The Editors*

Map Legend

Walk Route, paved		Swimming Pool	
Walk Route, unpaved		Swimming and Fishing Areas	
Interstate Highways		Boating Access	
Streets and Roads		River or Stream	
Hiking/Walking Trail		Waterfall	
Start/Finish of Loop Walk	S/F	Lake or Pond	
MetroLink Station	M	Park, Garden, or Wooded Area	
MetroLink Line		Spring	
Parking Area	P	Boundary, State Park or Institution	
Building		Interstate	00
Church or Cathedral	†	U.S. Highway	00
Restrooms, Male and Female		State and County Roads	00
Handicapped Access		Railroad	+++++
Food Vendor		Map Orientation	N
Picnic Area		Scale of Distance	0 0.5 1 Miles
Playground			
Athletic Field		Overlook or Point of Interest	
Tennis Courts			

Overview Map

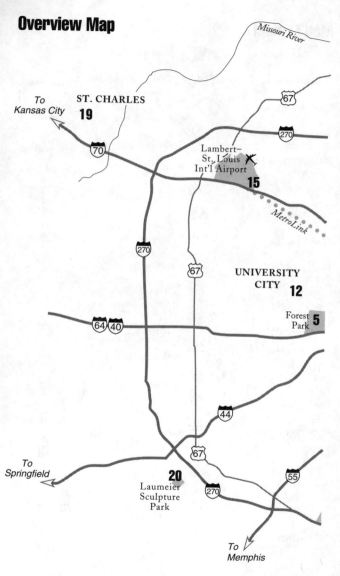

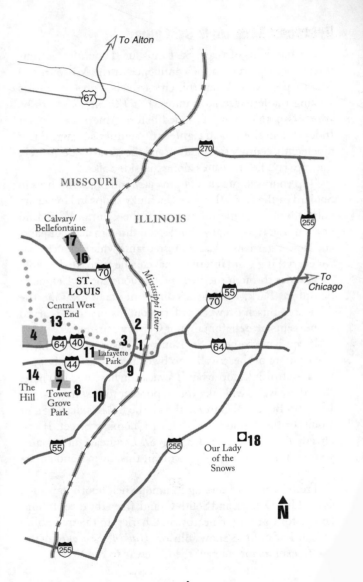

Preface: Come walk St. Louis

For hundreds of years, St. Louis lured countless adventurers and explorers to the confluence of the Missouri and Mississippi rivers. Today this city attracts scores of tourists seeking modern-day adventures. Let *Walking St. Louis* be your passport to a city founded before America's War for Independence. From an eighteenth-century street grid to a nineteenth-century train station and the ultra-modern Arch, this city lays her treasures along her sidewalks.

Tap your walking shoes to the jazz and blues rhythms in Soulard or the Loop. Explore the funky shops in University City; admire elegant, old homes in the Central West End or along Lafayette Square; and stroll through acres of parks and flower gardens. Walk to restaurants where you can savor everything from international cuisine to toasted ravioli.

Wander through the free and fabulous zoo or Laumeier Sculpture Park, sample a complimentary brew at the Anheuser-Busch Brewery, or ferret out history in the carved monuments of Bellefontaine or Calvary cemeteries.

If you have come to St. Louis on business, most likely one or more of these walks go by or near your hotel or are just a MetroLink stop away. If a vacation has lured you here, then these walks will take you to popular tourist haunts: the Missouri Botanical Garden, the Cathedral Basilica of Saint Louis, or the antique shops along Cherokee Street. If you already live in the area, *Walking St. Louis* can turn you or your visitors into sidewalk scouts in this diverse and entertaining city.

From Laclede's Landing to unique neighborhoods such as the Hill, Delmar, and South Grand; from the quaint shops and historic setting of nearby St. Charles; to the tranquility of Our Lady of the Snows Shrine, *Walking St. Louis* invites you to explore for yourself the Gateway to the West.

Introduction

Walking the streets and boulevards of a city can take you into its heart and give you a feel for its pulse and personality. From the sidewalk looking up, you can appreciate its architecture. From the sidewalk peeking in, you can find the quaint shops, local museums, and great eateries that give a city its charm and personality. From its nature paths, you can smell the flowers, glimpse the wildlife, gaze at a lake, or hear a creek gurgle. Only by walking can you get close enough to read the historical plaques and watch the people. When you walk a city, you get it all—adventure, scenery, local color, good exercise, and fun.

How to use this guide

We have designed this book so that you can easily find the walks that match your interests, time, and energy level. The Trip Planner is the first place you should look when deciding on a walk. This table will give you the basic information—a walk's distance, the estimated walking time, and the difficulty. The pictures or icons in the table also tell you specific things about the walk:

Every walk has something of interest, but this icon tells you that the route will have particular appeal to the shutterbug. So bring your camera. You will have great views of the city or the surrounding area, and you are likely to get some great scenic shots.

Somewhere along the route you will have the chance to get food or a beverage. You will have to glance through the walk description to determine where and wh⸢ kind of food and beverages are available. Walks that do ⸢ have the food icon probably are along nature trails ⸢ noncommercial areas of the city.

1

During your walk you will have the chance to shop. More detailed descriptions of the types of stores you will find can be found in the actual walk description.

This walk features something kids will enjoy seeing or doing—a park, zoo, museum, or play equipment. In most cases the walks that carry this icon are short and follow an easy, fairly level path. You know your young walking companions best. If your children are patient walkers who do not tire easily, then feel free to choose walks that are longer and harder. In fact, depending on a child's age and energy, most children can do any of the walks in this book. The icon only notes those walks we think they will especially enjoy.

Your path will take you primarily through urban areas. Buildings, small city parks, and paved paths are what you will see and pass.

You will pass through a large park or walk in a natural setting where you can see and enjoy nature.

The wheelchair icon means that the path is fully accessible. This walk would be easy for someone pushing a wheelchair or stroller. We have made every attempt to follow a high standard for accessibility. The icon means there are curb cuts or ramps along the entire route, plus a wheelchair-accessible bathroom somewhere along the way. The path is mostly or entirely paved, and ramps and unpaved surfaces are clearly described. If you use a wheelchair and have the ability to negotiate curbs and dirt paths or to wheel for longer distances and on uneven surfaces, you may want to skim the directions for the walks that do not carry this symbol. You may find other walks you will enjoy. If in doubt, the full text of the walk or call the contact source for advice.

Joggers also are likely to enjoy many of the walks in this book. All walks are easy and most have level routes and paved or smooth surfaces.

At the start of each walk chapter, you will find specific information describing the route and what you can expect on your walk:

General location: Here you will get the walk's general location in the city or within a specific area.

Special attractions: Look here to find the specific things you will pass. If this walk has museums, historic homes, restaurants, or wildlife, it will be noted here.

Difficulty: For this book, we have selected walking routes that an average person in reasonable health can complete easily. In most cases, you will be walking on flat surfaces with few, if any, hills. Your path will most likely be a maintained surface of concrete, asphalt, wood, or packed dirt. It will be easy to follow, and you will be only a block or so from a phone, other people, or businesses. If the walk is less than a mile, you may be able to walk comfortably in street shoes. If you are in doubt about whether you can manage a particular walk, read the description carefully or call the listed contact for more information.

Distance and estimated time: This gives the total distance of the walk. The time allotted for each walk is based on walking time only, which we have calculated at about 30 minutes per mile, a slow pace. Most people have no trouble walking a mile in half an hour, and people with some walking experience often walk a 20-minute mile. If the walk includes museums, shops, or restaurants, you may want to add sightseeing time to the estimate.

Services: Here you will find out if such things as restrooms, parking, refreshments, or information centers are availab' and where you are likely to find them.

3

Restrictions: The most often noted restriction regards pets, which almost always have to be leashed in a city. Most cities also have strict "pooper-scooper" laws, and they enforce them. Restrictions may also include the hours or days a museum or business is open, age requirements, or whether you can ride a bicycle on the path. If there is something you are not allowed to do on this walk, it will be noted here.

For more information: Each walk includes at least one contact source for you to call for more information. If an agency or business is named as a contact, you will find its phone number and address in Appendix B. This appendix also includes contact information for any business or agency mentioned anywhere in the book.

Getting started: Here you will find specific directions to the starting point. The majority of our walks are closed-loop walks, which means they begin and end at the same point. So you do not have to worry about finding your way back to your car or bus stop when your walk is over.

In those cities with excellent public transportation, it may be simple—and sometimes even more interesting—to finish a few walks somewhere other than the starting point. When this is the case, you will be provided with clear directions on how to take public transportation back to your starting point.

If a walk is not a closed-loop walk, this section will tell you where the walk ends. You will find the exact directions back to your starting point at the end of the walk's directions.

You may begin some downtown walks at any one of several hotels the walk passes. The directions will describe the route from the main starting point, but we will tell you if it s possible to join the route at other locations. If you are aying at a downtown hotel, it is likely that a walk passes in nt of or near your hotel's entrance.

Public transportation: Many cities have excellent transportation systems; others have limited services. If it is possible to take a bus or commuter train to the walk's starting point, you will find the bus or train noted here. You may also find some information about where the bus or train stops and how often and when it runs.

Overview: Every part of a city has a story to tell. Here is where you will find the story or stories about the people, neighborhoods, and history connected to your walk.

The walk

When you reach this point, you are ready to start walking. In this section you will find not only specific and detailed directions, but you will also learn more about the things you are passing. Those who want only the directions and none of the extras can find the straightforward directions by looking for the ➤.

What to wear

The best advice is to wear something comfortable. Leave behind anything that binds, pinches, rides up, falls down, slips off the shoulder, or comes undone. Otherwise, let common sense, the weather, and your own body tell you what to wear.

What to take

Be sure to take water. Strap a bottle to your fanny pack or tuck a small one in a pocket. If you are walking several miles with a dog, remember to take a small bowl so your pet can have a drink, too.

Carry some water even if you will be walking w' refreshments are available. Several small sips taken thr out a walk are more effective than one large drin' walk's end. Avoid drinks with caffeine or alcoh they deplete rather than replenish your body's fluids.

A fanny pack also comes in handy. It can hold your water as well as your keys, money, and sunglasses. It leaves your hands free to read your directions. If you will be gone for several hours and will walk where there are few or no services, you may want to carry a light backpack containing beverages and snacks.

Safety and street savvy

Mention a big city and many people immediately think of safety. Is it safe to walk there during the day? What about at night? Are there areas I should avoid?

You should use common sense whether you are walking in a small town or a big city, but safety does not have to be your overriding concern. American cities are enjoyable places, and if you follow some basic tips, you will find that they are also safe places.

Any safety mishap in a large city is likely to involve petty theft or vandalism. So, the biggest tip is simple: Do not tempt thieves. Purses dangling on shoulder straps or slung over your arm, wallets peeking out of pockets, arms burdened with packages, valuables on the car seat—all of these things attract the pickpocket, purse snatcher, or thief. If you look like you could easily be relieved of your possessions, you may be.

Do not carry a purse. Put your money in a money belt or tuck your wallet into a deep side pocket of your pants or skirt or in a fanny pack that rides over your hip or stomach. Lock your valuables in the trunk of your car before you park and leave for your walk. Protect your camera by wearing the strap across your chest, not just over your shoulder. Better yet, put your camera in a backpack.

You also will feel safer if you remember the following:

Be aware of your surroundings and the people near you.

6

- Avoid parks or other isolated places at night.
- Walk with others.
- Walk in well-lit and well-traveled areas.

The walks in this book were selected by people who had safety in mind. No walk will take you through a bad neighborhood or into an area of the city that is known to be dangerous. So relax and enjoy your walk.

Share the fun

We have tried to walk you to and through the best this city has to offer. But you may well discover other wonderful things—a fabulous bakery, a park tucked inside a neighborhood, a historic tidbit, or an interesting museum. Be sure to write to us care of Falcon Publishing and share your discovery. We would love to hear from you.

Walk name	Difficulty	Distance (miles)	Time	♿	🏙	🌳	⛲	📖	☕	📷
Downtown										
1. Jefferson National Expansion Memorial	easy	2	1 hr	✓	✓		✓	✓	✓	✓
2. Laclede's Landing	easy	.5	30 min	✓	✓		✓	✓	✓	
3. City Sights	easy	4.25	2.5 hrs	✓	✓		✓	✓	✓	✓
Forest Park										
4. Park Tour	easy	4	2 hrs	✓		✓	✓	✓	✓	✓
5. St. Louis Zoo	easy	1.5	1 hr	✓		✓	✓	✓	✓	✓
Tower Grove Park										
6. Missouri Botanical Garden	easy	2	1 hr	✓		✓	✓	✓	✓	✓
7. Park Tour	easy	2	1 hr	✓		✓	✓	✓	✓	
8. Grand South Grand	easy	1	30 min	✓	✓		✓	✓	✓	
St. Louis Neighborhoods										
9. Soulard	easy	2.5–4	1–3 hrs	✓	✓			✓	✓	
10. Cherokee Street	easy	1	30 min		✓			✓	✓	

	Difficulty	Distance	Time	Access	City setting	Nature setting	Good for kids	Shopping	Food	Bring camera
11. Lafayette Square	easy	0.75–1.25	30 min		✓		✓	✓	✓	✓
12. University City	easy	3.5	2 hrs		✓		✓	✓	✓	✓
13. Central West End	easy	4	2 hrs		✓			✓	✓	✓
14. The Hill	easy	1	30 min		✓				✓	✓
The All Day Tour										
15. The MetroLink Walk	easy	1–30	30 min+		✓		✓	✓	✓	✓
Historic Cemeteries										
16. Bellefontaine Cemetery	easy	3.5	2 hrs		✓	✓	✓		✓	✓
17. Calvary Cemetery	easy	2	1.5 hrs		✓	✓	✓			✓
In the Area										
18. Our Lady of the Snows Shrine	easy	2.5	1.5 hrs		✓	✓	✓		✓	✓
19. St. Charles	easy	2.3	1.5 hrs		✓		✓	✓	✓	✓
20. Laumeier Sculpture Park	easy	0.75–1	1 hr		✓	✓	✓			✓

the icons

Access	City setting	Nature setting	Good for kids	Shopping	Food	Bring camera

Meet St. Louis

Fast Facts

General
Time Zone: Central
Area Code: 314

Size
Missouri's second largest city after Kansas City
397,000 people
2.5 million people in metro area
61.4 square miles

Elevation
413 to 616 feet above sea level

Climate
Average yearly precipitation: 30 to 35 inches
Summer humidity: 80 to 90 percent
Maximum average temperature: 80-90 degrees
Minimum average temperature: 40 degrees

Getting there

Major highways
Interstates: 44, 55, 64, 70
Bypass routes: 170, 270, 255
U.S. highways: 40, 50, 67
State highways: 30, 100, 180, 340, 367

Airport service
Air Canada, American, America West, Continental, Delta, Northwest, Southwest, TWA, USAir, United

:l/bus service
:ntrak
:hound, Trailways

Major industries
Transportation, manufacturing, brewing, retailing, finance, construction, and recreation

Media
Television stations
ABC—Channel 30
CBS—Channel 4
Fox—Channel 30
NBC—Channel 5
PBS—Channel 9
Radio stations
KMOX 1120 AM—All-news/weather
KWMU 90.7 FM—National Public Radio
Newspaper
St. Louis Post Dispatch, morning daily

Recreation
More than 12,000 acres of public parks

Special annual events
Contact the St. Louis Convention and Visitors Commission to confirm dates and locations.

•February: Soulard Mardi Gras, Blueberry Hill's Elvis Birthday Celebration, Annual Orchid Show, Missouri WineFest

•March: Mid-America Jazz Festival, St. Patrick's Day Parade, Easter Egg Display at Our Lady of the Snows Shrine

•April: Annual Blueberry Hill Dart Tournament, Grand South Grand House Tour, Storytelling Festival

•May: Central West End House & Garden Tour, Laumeier Contemporary Art Fair, Lewis and Clark Rendezvous, Annie Malone Parade

- June: African Arts Festival
- July 4: Fair St. Louis
- July 14: Soulard Bastille Day
- August: Annual Japanese Festival, Goldenrod Ragtime Festival
- September: Big Muddy Blues Festival, Great Forest Park Balloon Race, Taste of St. Louis
- November-December: Brewery Lights Display, Shrine Way of Lights

In the Know

Weather

St. Louis has four distinct seasons. In the summer, the city's location between the Missouri and Mississippi rivers results in high humidity, which is often coupled with temperatures in the 90s. In July and August, the city steams, so bring light, breathable clothing.

Winters can feature everything from heavy snows, biting winds, and below-zero temperatures to days that are dry, mild, and sunny. Both winter-weather scenarios can happen in the same month or even the same week!

In the spring and fall, the city's many trees and shrubs sparkle with spring blooms or rich fall colors. These seasons bring moderate temperatures and especially beautiful and comfortable days for walking.

Because St. Louis's weather can be changeable, check your national weather forecast before packing for a trip or planning an outing.

Transportation

By car: If you drive into St. Louis, the first thing you will surely notice is the traffic. According to the St. Louis Convention and Visitors Commission, almost 90 percent of city visitors come by car. And with more than 2 million people living in and moving around the greater metro area, it is no wonder the highways are crowded.

Morning and evening rush hours are heavy and have a way of blending together. If you are traveling into the city, be prepared for the traffic to get heavier about 50 miles outside the city limits. On the Illinois side of the Mississippi River, the bridges into the city are jammed with cars during the morning rush hour, but the traffic lightens as you head out of the city into Illinois. Fortunately, St. Louis has a good highway system that keeps the traffic moving—most of the time. If you have not driven much or at all in St. Louis, do not let all those cars and green highway signs intimidate you. In no time, you will find yourself getting around easily and efficiently.

With its back against the Mississippi River, St. Louis grew outward from the river and along its banks. The major highways retrace these early supply routes. Almost every principal roadway either passes the Gateway Arch—the site where the city began—or heads directly into the downtown area.

The founding fathers laid out St. Louis in a grid. The streets start at the river and work their way west, so the numbers of the north-south streets get higher the farther you are from the river. Downtown's east-west Market Street divides the area north to south, so the City Museum at 701 North 15th Street is about fifteen blocks west of the river and about seven blocks north of Market.

By bus: Bi-State Transit, the public bus system for the St Louis area, offers service on the Missouri and Illinois sid of the Mississippi River. Most buses start and end at downtown terminal, and most have wheelchair lifts. many cities, it is easy to get around by bus within t limits but more challenging if you want to get t the suburbs. Bi-State also offers "Call-A-Ride," which is open to anyone traveling from areas not readily served by Bi-State buses. Call-A-Ride-Plus offers transportation to those with disabilities who are registered with the service.

Greyhound and Trailways are the commercial bus lines that serve the city.

By air: St. Louis is within a four-hour flight of all major U.S. cities, and almost one dozen airlines come into Lambert-St. Louis International Airport, about 15 miles northwest of downtown. The MetroLink, the city's light-rail system, goes to the airport, so it is possible to get into the city in about thirty minutes for as little as one dollar per person. A taxi ride from Lambert to downtown will cost about twenty dollars and may take around an hour—depending on traffic.

By train: Amtrak has two passenger stations—one in downtown St. Louis and another in the nearby suburb of Kirkwood.

Safety

Midwestern cities such as St. Louis generally are friendlier and more hospitable than those on either coast. But St. Louis is a big city with a big-city crime rate. Let common sense guide you as you stroll this city. It may help to remember that we selected these particular walks because they offer enjoyable walking experiences in lively and interesting areas that are also safe.

In general, it is best to walk during daylight so you can read your maps, enjoy the sights, and watch for holes and uneven surfaces on the path. You should undertake some lks, such as Forest Park and Tower Grove Park, only during the day.

ll, nice evenings invite people to walk, and well-lit isy with tourists and night activities provide safe walkers. Laclede's Landing, Delmar Boulevard's

1 4

Loop, Soulard, and the Central West End, for example, bustle with activity well into the early morning hours. Evening walks in these areas are both safe and delightful.

St. Louis's larger downtown area, however, is much less busy at night. The Gateway Arch and Union Station may stay active—especially in warmer weather—but the areas around Busch Stadium, the TWA Dome, and the streets between Laclede's Landing and the downtown hotels most often will be quiet. Although well lit and well traveled, the downtown streets will not feel as welcoming at night. Even if no danger lurks, you may feel uneasy.

If you find yourself walking after dark downtown or off the beaten path in Soulard, University City, Lafayette Square, or South Grand, avoid alleyways, parks, and parking lots. When possible, walk with other people and choose well-lit thoroughfares.

For a general review of city safety information, read the tips on page 6, and enjoy your walks.

The story of St. Louis

People have walked the land in and around St. Louis since about 20,000 B.C. Leaving only mounds of earth as proof of their existence, these early inhabitants gave St. Louis one of its first nicknames—Mound City. Generations later, the Missouri, Osage, Kansas, Otoe, Iowa, and Omaha Indians migrated to the land between the two great rivers——the Missouri and the Mississippi. Here the soil was rich, the game and fur-bearing animals plentiful, and travel faster on the swiftly flowing rivers.

The Spaniards traveled through the Midwest in the mid-1500s. But it was the French fur trappers and missionaries navigating the Mississippi River south from Canada in the 1600s who opened the land to Europeans. When the French explorer La Salle traveled the Mississippi from just north of St. Louis all the way to the Gulf of Mexico, he claimed all the land watered by the mighty river for King Louis XIV of France. He christened the territory Louisiana.

In 1763, when St. Louis founding father Pierre Laclède pointed his boat toward the bluffs below what is now Laclede's Landing, France and her business allies had already established New Orleans and a vast trading network with trappers and Indians. Laclède wanted a convenient and protected spot along the Mississippi River where he could build a successful fur-trading center.

Impressed by this site's central location, its abundant timber and building stone, fresh water, and enough elevation to protect it from flooding, Laclède was said to have announced that this land "might become, hereafter, one of the finest cities." Laclède gave the job of establishing the settlement to Auguste Chouteau, the fourteen-year-old son of Madame Marie Thérèse Chouteau and half-brother to the ir children of Laclède and Marie Thérèse.

Obviously not an ordinary teenager, but rather an urban planning prodigy, Auguste is considered the city's co-founder. He supervised not only the initial construction of the fur post, but also Laclède's stone house and the town's layout. The design included a public market square, a church block, and common lands to the west for farming and grazing.

Laclède named the town St. Louis after Crusader King Saint Louis IX, the patron saint of King Louis XV—the reigning French monarch. He did not know that two years earlier France had secretly given her lands west of the Mississippi to Spain. In 1800, Napoleon recovered the land for France, but in a few years he would sell it again—this time to a young United States for $15 million.

The politics of kings and generals mattered little to the Creoles who came from Canada and the Gulf to make a life in St. Louis. They spoke French; their social and business ties were to France, New Orleans, and Quebec. In the 1700s, St. Louis reflected the customs, gaiety, and tolerance associated with French culture.

In 1804, the Louisiana Purchase—the world's largest real estate deal—converted St. Louis from a French to a U.S. city. Meriwether Lewis and William Clark, who were in St. Louis to begin their celebrated exploration of the new lands, witnessed the lowering of the French flag—the last to ever fly in North America—and the raising of the American. The Gateway to the West was about to open, and with it would come a wave of gold seekers, settlers, and adventurers. By the 1900s, St. Louis would be the fourth largest city in the nation.

In 1821, Missouri entered the Union as a slave state. Louisans strongly felt the tensions that eventually w divide the North and South. Although the city sa one skirmish, its proximity to the South and its bor status hurt its trading opportunities. Rail and commercial activity headed north to Chicago. Increased western migration after the war brought renewed activity, but by the turn of the century, St. Louis was in a slump.

The Louisiana Purchase Exposition—more commonly known as the 1904 World's Fair—revived St. Louis's spirits and brought the city well-deserved accolades. City residents used every ounce of community spirit and available cash to create a fair that astounded people with its beauty and sophistication. It was, many have said, the city's crowning moment.

For the first half of the 1900s, St. Louis seemed to prefer to rest on its fair laurels rather than continue to rebuild a city that had clearly started to show its age. Urban blight and urban flight were bringing a once vital city to ruin.

As the beauty of modern St. Louis shows, the city did not crumble. Instead, it was renewed and restored. The Jefferson National Expansion Memorial, with its gleaming Arch resting on Laclède's home site; Busch Stadium; the St. Louis Centre; and reclaimed and refurbished neighborhoods brought people back to the city, not only to visit, but also to live. Visitors now come by the millions to walk the beautifully landscaped parks, catch a baseball game at Busch Stadium, enjoy the city's free museums and zoo, or catch the strains of St. Louis blues. This restored and vital old river town—first built by a few hardy Frenchmen in pursuit of personal wealth—still maintains its rightful place as this country's historic gateway to the West.

walk 1

Jefferson National Expansion Memorial

General location: At the Gateway Arch.

Special attractions: The arch, museums, views of the river and downtown skyline, an urban forest, and the historic Old Courthouse.

Difficulty rating: Easy, flat, entirely on paved surfaces, a great path for joggers.

Distance: 2 miles.

Estimated time: 1 hour.

Services: Bathrooms, including wheelchair-accessible one are in the memorial's lower level, where you will also fi pop machines and a gift shop. For restaurants go to ne Laclede's Landing or into the Admiral Casino.

19

Jefferson National Expansion Memorial

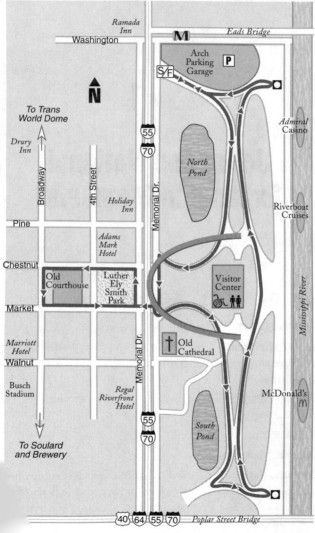

Restrictions: The arch's observation area is not wheelchair-accessible. Dogs must be leashed and cannot be left unattended on park grounds or tied to trees or railings. Except for dogs assisting people with disabilities, dogs are not allowed inside park buildings. No swimming or wading in the reflection ponds.

For more information: Contact the Jefferson National Expansion Memorial or the St. Louis Convention and Visitors Commission.

Getting started: All roads heading downtown seem eventually to lead to the Gateway Arch. Interstates 44, 55, 64, and 70 merge just south of Jefferson National Expansion Park, so follow any of the interstates toward downtown and watch for the signs directing you to the arch and the parking garage. You will enter the garage off Washington Street, just east of Memorial Drive. The garage charges a modest fee.

This walk starts at the edge of the parking garage, located between the arch and Laclede's Landing. Depending on how you approach the Gateway Arch, however, you can pick up this closed-looped path in one of several spots: any of the park's four sidewalk entrances off Memorial Drive, the sidewalk next to the Old Courthouse, or the upper level of the Arch Parking Garage, which is the best choice for those in wheelchairs or pushing strollers. Check the map on page 20 to find the spot where you can pick up the path. If you are driving an RV, you can park in a pay lot under the Poplar Street Bridge, at the south end of the Gateway Arch grounds.

This walk is also close to several downtown hotels. Locate your hotel on the map to determine where you go t start this walk.

Public transportation: The MetroLink stops at Laclede's L ing, which is just north of the Jefferson Nat

Expansion Park and just across Washington from where this walk starts. Several buses also stop near or at the Gateway Arch and the Old Courthouse. Contact the Bi-State Transit Information Center to find the bus most convenient for you.

Overview: As Barringer Fifield so aptly notes in his book *Seeing Saint Louis*, "The Arch is where everything comes together. The improbably stainless steel flourish unites not only earth and sky, land and water, east and west, but also St. Louis's past and present, its challenges and responses. Here is where the city begins. . . ."

This ribbon of steel is as evocative of St. Louis as the Eiffel Tour is of Paris or the Statue of Liberty of New York. When you come to the arch, you come to the starting point of St. Louis's history. When you stand beneath it, you stand where founding father Pierre Laclède once stood. When you ride to the top of the arch, you survey the land that greeted fur trappers, explorers, missionaries, immigrants, and pioneers heading West.

As a memorial, this 22-acre park pays tribute to Thomas Jefferson, who finalized the Louisiana Purchase; to Meriwether Lewis and William Clark, who mapped and explored the new territory; to the settlers who built the city's first homes and businesses on this spot; to the pioneers who sweated and muscled the West into existence; and to the Mississippi and Missouri rivers, which enabled St. Louis to prosper.

The arch and its grounds were thirty years in the planning and building. Franklin D. Roosevelt was president when the Jefferson National Expansion Memorial Association was formed; Lyndon B. Johnson was president when the park and arch were "Dedicated to the people of the United States" May 25, 1968.

In addition to the arch, the grounds include the Old Courthouse, the building with the dome on the other side of Memorial Drive; the Museum of Westward Expansion, located under the arch; and the Arch Visitor Center. This center includes three information kiosks, which also give information on accessibility; the tram waiting area; the museum gift shop; and two theaters, one showing the Academy Award-nominated film *Monument to the Dream* and

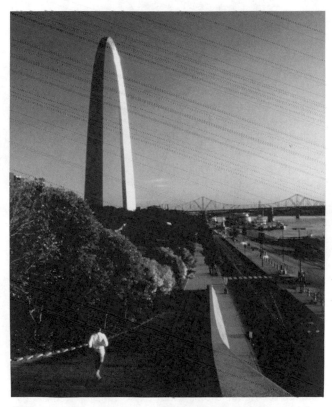

Walkers and joggers enjoy three miles of paths at the Jefferson National Expansion Memorial. PHOTO COURTESY OF ST. LOUIS CONVENTION AND VISITORS COMMISSION.

the other *The Great American West*, which is shown on a several-stories-tall screen. This walk will take you to all these places.

of interest

The Gateway Arch

In the late 1940s, Eero Saarinen, a Finnish-born architect, designed the arch using the shape of a weighted catenary curve. He died of brain cancer in 1961, four years before the arch was completed. During his career he worked on such projects as TWA's terminal in New York and Dulles International Airport outside Washington, D.C. However, the arch remains his most memorable work.

At 630 feet, the arch is the tallest man-made monument in the United States. It is 75 feet taller than the Washington Monument and twice as tall as the Statue of Liberty. But it is smaller than the Eiffel Tower (984 feet) and just half the size of New York's Empire State Building.

With an outer layer of shiny stainless steel, the arch mirrors what surrounds it, catching and reflecting the color of blue skies or gray thunderheads, the blazing sun or midnight moon, the first light of dawn or the shimmer of city lights at night. Only the light coming from its surroundings illuminates it, so its appearance changes with the time of day and weather. It is no wonder that to those who see it often, the arch appears to have a life of its own.

On this walk you will see the arch from every side. As you watch it, watch the people who have come to see and experience this graceful formation. Some stand under it and crane their necks upward; others stand close to sense its mass and heat; still others run their hands along its metal flanks to feel its strength. On a windy day as the clouds billow by, the arch appears to glide in rhythm with the sky. Before your walk is over, be sure that you, too, touch the arch.

of interest

Arch Facts

Designer: Eero Saarinen
Completed: October 28, 1965
Cost: $13 million
Height: 630 feet, or about 63 stories
Span: 630 feet at ground level
Weight: 43,000 tons
Foundation: 60 feet deep
Sway: Half inch to an inch in 20 mph wind
Visitors: 65 million since 1967
      4.5 million yearly
      15,000-30,000 a day in the summer,
      with 5,500 of those going to the top

The walk

➤Start this walk at the park's northwest corner, near the intersection of Washington Street and Memorial Drive, at the sign announcing this national park as the Jefferson National Expansion Memorial. This is, by the way, the first national park placed within a city.

The park is closed between 11 p.m. and 6 a.m. For safety reasons, please do not walk in the park after hours. When it is open, however, the park is well populated and well lit with many street lamps.

➤At the park sign, walk into this tree-lined area. The park contains almost three thousand trees, many of them rosehill ash. You will be walking toward the Mississippi River and away from downtown. To your right you will see the North Pond, and soon you will see the parking lot's upper-level entrance into the park.

of interest

Tram tips

If you are claustrophobic, skip the tram and visit one of the kiosks in the visitor center for a video "trip to the top." Those going up will join four other people for a four-minute ride in a small capsule that resembles a space module. Do not let the periodic jolts startle you.

On a clear day, you can see about thirty miles from the top; on windy days, you may feel a slight sway. On hot days, the observatory heats up; the temperature at the top is posted in the visitor center where you buy your tickets.

Speaking of tickets: You buy tickets for a specific ascent time. On busy days—which are most days in the summer and holidays—tickets may be sold out two to three hours or more ahead. You might want to buy your tickets and then take your walk or come early in the morning before the crowds.

When you are finished at the top, you will wait only a short time for your three-minute descent. Remember, there are no restrooms in the observatory.

➤Follow the path as it curves to your right. The lawn slopes down to the pond, where you might see some ducks or geese. As you walk along on this side of the park, you will get some great views of the city on your right and the river on your left. Those mighty waters are what started the St. Louis story and made this city a reality.

You will find benches and plenty of trash cans along the park pathways. This spot is perfect for a light picnic lunch. You can eat a sandwich and enjoy the views.

At the base of the arch's north leg, take the trail that veers to your right, away from the river and toward downtown.

You will have a stunning view of the Old Courthouse at the top of this path. You are now walking toward Memorial Drive. The city is spread out in front of you.

➤At Memorial Drive, turn left and walk to Market Street, which will come up on your right.

➤Cross Memorial Drive at Market, being careful to cross at the crosswalk and with the lights. At the corner of Memorial Drive and Market, you will see a sign for the Jefferson National Expansion Memorial. You are now in the part of the national park that includes the Old Courthouse.

➤Turn right after crossing Memorial Drive and walk in front of the courthouse. Look to your right to catch great views of the arch. The Luther Ely Smith Park is to your left. Smith was a tireless proponent of the Jefferson National Expansion Memorial. In the summer, these gardens are filled with red canna.

➤Turn left at Chestnut.

➤At 4th Street and Chestnut, cross 4th.

➤Continue one block to Broadway and turn left. You are now in front of the historic Old Courthouse. If the courthouse is open, take a moment and go inside. Some historic people, including the slave Dred Scott, have walked the steps you are now walking. If you are using a wheelchair, the stair lift is on this side. Press the bell for service.

➤Leave the courthouse through the same door you entered.

➤At the bottom of the steps, turn left and go to Market.

➤Turn left at Market and go to Memorial Drive.

➤Cross Memorial Drive in the crosswalk and with the lights.

➤Once across Memorial, pick up the park path as it heads toward the river. Here you will get a sense of the immense

of interest

The Old Courthouse

Framed by the Gateway Arch, the Old Courthouse is one of the downtown's oldest buildings; it dates back to the 1820s. It is made of cold stone, but its history runs hot with emotion.

For the pioneers heading West, the courthouse was a place of excitement, for here they met up with their wagon trains. For slaves, the courthouse meant sorrow, for slave auctions were held on the east steps. Occasionally, slave owners came to the courthouse to manumit, or free, their slaves. Ulysses S. Grant freed his one and only slave here in 1859.

Dred Scott, the area's most renowned slave, came in 1846 to sue for freedom. Having lived briefly in two free states, he argued he could not be returned to bondage in Missouri. The lower court agreed, but not the Missouri Supreme Court. Scott appealed to the U.S. Supreme Court and lost. The court's ruling nullified the Missouri Compromise, which had kept a precarious peace between the North and South. Slavery became legal in every U.S. territory, and the nation moved closer to war.

The first-floor courtroom where Scott's case was heard disappeared during remodeling. The first floor now houses the museum galleries, restrooms, gift shop, and the rotunda from which you can see the dome frescoes. The second floor, which is not accessible by wheelchair, has restored courtrooms.

This Greek Revival building was deeded to the National Park Service in 1940 and restored in the mid-1980s. Catch a view of the city from the dome's observation deck. Designed by William Rumbold, the dome is a year older than the one on the U.S. Capitol in Washington, D.C. The building also offers audio-tours and ranger-guided tours. Contact the Jefferson National Expansion Memorial for information on tours, trial reenactments, and special programs.

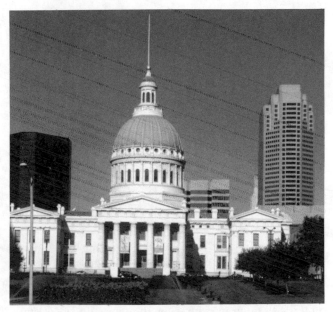

The iron dome of the Old Courthouse is thought to have inspired the Capitol dome in Washington, D.C.

size of the arch as it stretches over your head. Again you will get a good view of the Mississippi River. Depending on the time of year, you may see active barge traffic, because the Mississippi is a major grain highway.

➤Walk toward the south leg of the arch.

➤Follow the path as it curves to your right. The South Pond will come up on your right as you walk through this corridor of trees. At the southernmost point of this path, the trail divides. One branch leaves the park and heads downtown and the other goes left toward the river.

➤Take the path to your left. The trail will form a U that takes you back into the park and toward the arch. As you walk toward the river, you will notice a plaza with an overlook. Walk to its edge.

This observation plaza, known as the Lewis Overlook, is one of two that gives you a view of the river. The other, the Clark Overlook, is at the north end of the park. To your right is the Poplar Street Bridge. To your left, you will see stairs that go down toward the riverboats and the riverfront walk. A floating McDonald's restaurant—the first in the nation—shares the waterfront with other boats, which offer gambling, dinner dances, extended river trips, and narrated one-hour excursion cruises. Check Appendix B for information on these boats.

➤Return to the park path and head to your right toward the south leg of the arch. As you stand at the arch and look toward the city, you can see the Old Cathedral and the courthouse dome. If you want to stop by the arch's visitor center, gift shop, restrooms, or the Museum of Western Expansion, or see one of the two movies, or take a tram ride, follow the stairs or incline that leads you under the arch. You will find another entrance at the arch's north leg.

➤After your adventure under and perhaps atop the arch, continue on the trail that leads between the river and the arch. This trail will give you an opportunity to visit the Clark Overlook if you want another view of the river.

➤If you parked in the upper level of the parking garage, return to your car. If you parked on the lower level, on the street, or in a Laclede's Landing parking lot, follow the path around the parking garage and out of the park.

walk 2
Laclede's Landing

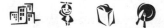

General location: Beside the Mississippi River, just north of the Gateway Arch, between the Eads and Dr. Martin Luther King bridges.

Special attractions: Popular music venues and restaurants, historic buildings, museums, nineteenth-century architecture, carriage rides. The trendiest stop is the Planet Hollywood restaurant.

Difficulty rating: Easy, but watch your footing on the uneven cobblestone streets.

Distance: Half a mile.

Estimated time: 30 minutes.

Services: Restaurants and bars. You will find something open from about 8 a.m. to the wee hours.

Restrictions: People pushing strollers will find the path

Laclede's Landing

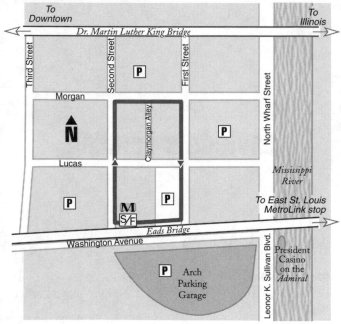

bumpy. It is best to leave your dog at home; heavy pedestrian traffic, horse-drawn carriages, and all-paved surfaces make this an unpleasant trek for four-footed walkers.

For more information: Contact the St. Louis Convention and Visitors Commission.

Getting started: This walk starts at the MetroLink Station for Laclede's Landing. The station is directly across the street from the entrance to the arch parking garage. All of the interstates coming into the downtown—I-44, I-55, I-64, and I-70—will take you to Laclede's Landing. Interstates 55 and 70 go directly past the arch and the Landing: take

Exit 250B onto Memorial Drive. If you are taking Interstates 44 or 64, watch for signs for I-55.

When you are close to the arch, you will see signs that direct you to the arch parking garage. You will enter the garage from Washington Avenue just east of Memorial Drive. The parking lot is large and the prices reasonable. The Laclede's area has parking space for 5,000 cars, so you are sure to find a spot.

This walk is also close to several downtown hotels. If you are staying at the Embassy Suites, walk straight south toward the Landing to the MetroLink stop. If your hotel is on either side of Washington Avenue, then take Washington toward the river. Look for the MetroLink stop just under Eads Bridge.

Public transportation: The MetroLink stops at Laclede's Landing. Several buses also go to the Landing and the nearby arch. Contact the Bi-State Transit Information Center to find the bus most convenient for you.

Overview: St. Louis's original settlement began in the area occupied by the Gateway Arch and the wharf area known as Laclede's Landing. Those early buildings and streets were cleared to make room for the park, so these 1850s warehouses and streets are all that remain of the city's oldest area. Here you will walk St. Louis as its early settlers walked it, on cobblestones and along narrow streets that are part of a grid laid out by founder Pierre Laclède in the late 1700s.

The original buildings in this nine-block historic district are gone. Some were made of stone; most, however, were constructed of upright logs covered with whitewash. But the wrought-iron street lamps and warehouses, some still displaying their decorative ironwork, capture what riverboat crews and passengers would have seen when they disembarked in the mid-1800s.

This wharf area once teemed with commerce. Crews unloaded tobacco, cotton, fur, and other goods into these warehouses. Today this carefully restored district teems with tourists and conventioneers. The warehouses have found new life as nightclubs, restaurants, office buildings, and shops.

Popular with the lunch crowd during the day, Laclede's Landing really comes alive at night. Strains of jazz, blues, ragtime, reggae and rock-n-roll float through the streets, entertaining both outdoor diners and strollers. The restaurants, nightclubs, and the President Casino on the *Admiral*—docked at the river—keep the area bustling into the wee hours.

The activity and crowds make this small district a safe place to walk both day and night. Each time of the day offers its own special charm.

The walk

➤Turn right when you exit the MetroLink. You are on Second Street, which is part of the street Laclède christened La Rue d'Eglise because it led to the settlement's first church. The cobblestone streets and red-brick sidewalks will accompany you throughout this short walk.

Along this 600 block you will find Kennedy's Restaurant and Bar. Planet Hollywood is a block to the left.

➤Cross Lucas Avenue and continue on Second.

When you cross Lucas, look to your left for a view of the Trans World Dome. Along this 700 block, on this side of the street, you will find Victoria's Kitchen and Ice Creamery and Jake's Steak House. Across the street is Hannegan's Restaurant and Pub and the Morgan Street Brewery.

Hannegan's dining room is a replica of the U.S. Senate Dining Room. In nice weather, it provides outdoor dining, and jazz groups play regularly. The Morgan Street Brewery offers patio dining and brewery tours in the Landing's oldest building.

At the end of this block, just as you approach the corner, you will find a vest-pocket park dedicated to Francis A. Mesker, an immigrant from Holland. Mesker sold metalware along the river, some of it similar to the ironwork that decorates the warehouses.

The sheltered garden, with its flowers and fountain, is reminiscent of the tiny garden spots you find in New Orleans or European cities and contributes to this area's distinctive Old World charm.

➤Turn right at the corner of Morgan and Second.

Note the large, four-faced clock across the street. But do not set your watch by it, for it is now purely decorative.

Across the street at 801 North Second Street, you will find the free National Video Game and Coin-Op Museum. It includes the first video game—Computer Space—plus more than seventy other landmark games. Step inside and see how pinball machines were invented or play classic video games like Pong, Pac-Man, and Donkey Kong.

Along Morgan, you may find horse-drawn carriages waiting to take you for a spin around the district. As you walk this block, look for the opening between the buildings that comes up on your right. This is Claymorgan Alley. From here you can get an interesting view of the arch and can pick up the strains of music coming from the bars and restaurants that open onto the alleyway. The next street is First Street—or Laclède's Le Grande Rue.

➤Go to First Street and turn right. In this area you will find bars and restaurants offering nightly music, family restaurants like the Old Spaghetti Factory, and the Royal Dumpe Dinner Theater where the Royal Dumplings put on family theater.

3 5

of interest

The Eads Bridge

The Eads, the world's first steel truss bridge, was built by James Buchanan Eads, a cousin to President James Buchanan. When it opened in May 1874, it was the first bridge in St. Louis to cross the Mississippi River, and more than 20,000 walkers paid five cents for the privilege of being among the first to walk its upper deck. Trains traveled its lower deck, and the Eads was the first bridge to take trains across the Mississippi River. Today the MetroLink crosses into East St. Louis, Illinois, via this bridge, making the Eads the oldest bridge still in use across the Mississippi River.

At #727 you will find the Dental Health Theater, the only museum in the country devoted to dental hygiene. Puppets, a film, and interesting props teach children how to take care of their teeth. The museum and programs are free, but you must make reservations. The building, once a tobacco factory, displays the decorative ironwork that was once common in the area.

As you walk south on First Street, take a moment to appreciate the Eads Bridge.

➤Cross Lucas Avenue. The parking lot at the corner of Lucas and First posts a sign for the *Admiral*, once the largest river excursion boat in the country and a great place for lunch. This pleasure boat now houses a casino and is permanently moored at the river just below the Landing. If you visit the casino and have parked in one of the Landing's lots, your parking is free.

➤Go under the Eads and turn right on Washington.

➤Return to the MetroLink station and the end of this walk.

walk 3
City Sights

General location: West of the Gateway Arch, in the heart of downtown.

Special attractions: The Gateway Arch and Mississippi River, historic sites, picturesque views, restored Union Station, great shopping, varied architecture, museums, Busch Stadium.

Difficulty rating: Easy, primarily flat, all on paved surfaces; one long stairway to the arch.

Distance: 4.25 miles.

Estimated time: 2.5 hours.

Services: Many restaurants and stores on this walk, and a few museums.

Restrictions: Dogs must be leashed and their droppings picked up. Dogs not allowed in Union Station or other buildings.

City Sights

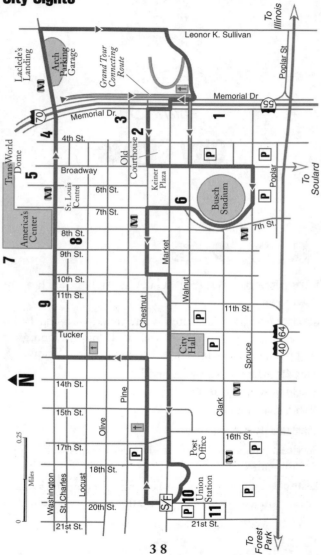

Hotels
1 Regal Riverfront
2 Adams Mark Hotel
3 Holiday Inn
4 Days Inn
5 Drury Inn
6 Marriot Pavilion Hotel
7 Holiday Inn
8 Mayfair Hotel
9 Days Inn
10 Hyatt Regency
11 Drury Inn

For more information: Contact the St. Louis Convention and Visitors Commission, the Jefferson National Expansion Memorial, or Union Station, depending on your question.

Getting started: This walk begins at Union Station, which is on Market Street between 18th and 20th streets. The station is less than one mile from all the interstates serving the city: I-44, I-55, I-70, and I-64/40. Interstate 64/40, however, passes closest to the station, with exits for 14th Street and for Market. Once on Market, follow the signs for Union Station. The station has a large parking lot, and you might find metered parking on the street.

You can also begin this walk from several downtown locations, including the MetroLink stops at the Convention Center, Laclede's Landing, 8th and Pine, or Busch Stadium. You can also start at the St. Louis Visitors Center at the corner of 7th and Washington. Tourists staying in one of the downtown hotels may find that this walk passes by or near their hotel's front door. Look at the map and find where you can pick up this walk's path.

Public transportation: The MetroLink, which offers convenient transportation in the downtown area, stops at Union Station. If you are coming into the downtown area, contact Bi-State Transit for the bus routes most convenient to you.

Overview: This walk lets you savor the many attractions that attract people to St. Louis—the arch, the Mississippi River, Busch Stadium, the Old Cathedral, Christ Church Cathedral, and Union Station, which is a vacation spot in itself. This sidewalk journey through the city's core gives walkers a variety of things to see and do, plus pleasing views of St. Louis sights. If you have not yet explored the Jefferson National Expansion Memorial or the Old Courthouse, now is the time to do it.

The walk

➤This walk starts at the corner of 20th and Market streets in front of Union Station.

➤Cross Market with the light. After you cross, look toward the river to catch a view of the arch curving over the downtown area.

➤Walk one block to Chestnut Street and turn right. Chances are you will not see a street sign for Chestnut. But Chestnut is the first street after Market. Union Station and Aloe Plaza's dramatic fountain display will be on your right as you walk east on Chestnut.

When the fountain's sculptures were unveiled in 1941, *The Meeting of the Waters* disturbed many St. Louisans. They were uncomfortable with Carl Milles's portrayal of the Mississippi River as a nude young man, of the Missouri River as a nude young woman, and of his obvious suggestion that the waters coupled in St. Louis. Today, however, this joyous fountain with its playful, mythological characters is a favorite landmark. If you are near Union Station on a pleasant evening, come and stand where you are now. The fountain lit up against the backdrop of the station will be an image you will long remember.

➤Continue east on Chestnut. Take a moment to appreciate this view of Union Station with its red roof, flags, and castlelike details. In warm weather, the flowering gardens add to its charm.

You will follow Chestnut to 13th Street and will see many architecturally interesting buildings along this grand boulevard.

The green space dividing Chestnut and Market is filled with trees, flower gardens, picnic tables, and benches.

At 18th and Market streets, directly east of Union Station, is the U.S. Post Office. Completed in 1937, it houses fresco murals depicting the history of St. Louis.

Coming up on your left at 16th and Chestnut streets you will pass St. John's Catholic Church. Built in 1860, it was the diocese's cathedral after the Civil War.

Off to your right at 15th Street is Kiel Auditorium with its distinctive columns. The statue in front is of Johann Schiller, a German dramatist. Behind the auditorium you can catch the rounded roof of the Kiel Center, a 20,000-seat sports arena and home to the Blues and the Ambush, the city's professional hockey and soccer teams, respectively.

When you cross 14th Street, you will get a better view of the Soldiers Memorial, built in the 1930s. Its two museum rooms are connected by an open area with a granite memorial to the dead of World War I. Facing Market at 14th are the Municipal Courts. Just beyond that is City Hall, which is a copy of Hôtel de Ville, Paris's city hall.

At 13th Street, look up and a little to your right and find the building with a temple perched on its top. This is the Civil Courts Building at 12th and Market. The temple is a replica of the tomb of King Mausolus and was built around 350 B.C. Mausolus's tomb was counted among the Seven Wonders of the Ancient World; the word mausoleum comes from his name. Directly across the street from the Civil Courts Buildings is the striking U.S. Court and Customs House, which was completed in 1934.

➤Cross 13th Street and turn left. You will walk along this side of 13th to Washington Street. Be careful as you cross the intersections between here and Washington, for these streets only have stop signs. Ahead of you and across the street to your left is the St. Louis Public Library. In front of you on your side of Chestnut is Christ Church Cathedral, the seat of the Episcopal Diocese.

The library at 1301 Olive Street, in Italian Renaissance style, was built in 1913 for $1.5 million. Andrew Carnegie covered almost half the costs. If the library is open, you may want to step inside to appreciate the lovely architectural detailing. Michelangelo's ceiling in Florence's Laurentian Library has been re-created here.

Christ Church Cathedral is an exceptional example of English Gothic architecture. Dedicated in 1867, after the Civil War had interrupted construction, the cathedral was home to the only Episcopal parish west of the Mississippi River. Step inside and view the stained glass windows, the altar, and the dramatic reredos, or wall behind the altar, which is filled with statuary. Both the altar and its backdrop were carved in England from stone taken from the famous quarries of Caen, France.

➤At Washington Street, turn right. You will stay on the south side of Washington for several blocks until you reach the promenade that runs along the Mississippi River. If you want to visit the City Museum—dinosaur remains, aquarium, caves, trains, and more—go two blocks to your left, then return to this spot.

Between 13th and 9th Streets you will walk through a part of the city's old warehouse district. With the river just down the street, this area was a natural storage and distribution center at the turn of the century. Many of the old warehouses have been refitted into office spaces. Just past the intersection of 9th and Washington, stop and closely examine the east side of the Lennox. The architectural details on this side are a trompe l'oeil. Can you spot the gentleman destined to forever take in a balcony view of the city?

The America's Center, one of the largest convention centers in the country, is coming up on your left. This complex

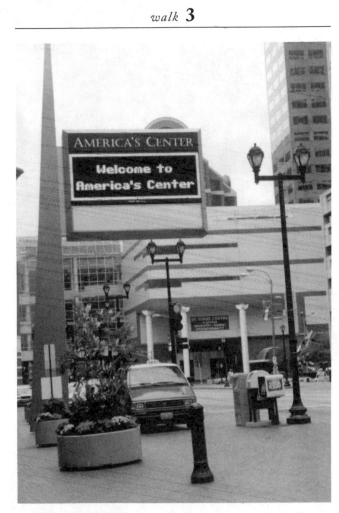

The America's Center and the white and green striped St. Louis Centre are cornerstones of the city's revitalization efforts.

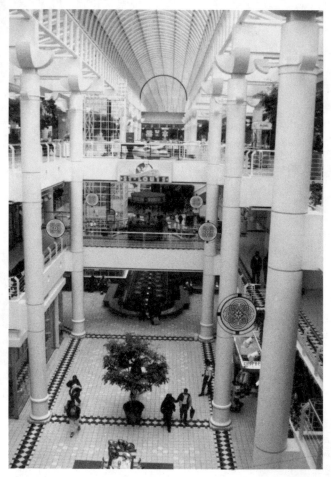

The St. Louis Centre is filled with shops, offices, and, on its top level, a food court.

includes the Cervantes Convention Center, with its exhibition halls, and the Trans World Dome Stadium, home of the NFL St. Louis Rams. You will get a better view of the dome when you reach the intersection of Broadway and Washington. The dome will be off to your left.

If you want tourist information, stop at the St. Louis Visitors Center. The center is across Washington Street in the America's Center, and its entrance is at the corner of 7th and Washington. The white and green-striped building ahead of you is the St. Louis Centre, a four-tier, indoor shopping mall that connects two major department stores: Famous-Barr and Dillards. When it opened in 1985, it was the largest enclosed urban shopping mall in the country. Its food court and restrooms are on the fourth floor.

At street level, just inside the center's 7th and Washington entrance, you will find the transit system's Metro Ride store. Its friendly staff can help you get anywhere in the city via public transportation. At the center's northeast entrance, you will find a MetroLink stop.

➤Continue on Washington, carefully crossing the next few busy intersections with the lights. When you have crossed Memorial Drive, continue on Washington toward the river. The multi-level arch parking garage is coming up on your right; Laclede's Landing will be to your left.

Walk 2, which begins on page 31, starts at the MetroLink stop and goes through Laclede's Landing. The stop is across the street on Second Street, just under the Eads Bridge. Walk 1, which begins on page 19, takes in the Jefferson National Expansion Memorial. That walk starts at the national park sign that appears on your right as you approach the parking garage.

➤Continue toward the river. From this vantage, you get a good sidewalk view of the Eads Bridge, which is mentioned on page 36.

➤At Leonor K. Sullivan Boulevard, turn right and walk along the promenade. This boulevard is named for the St. Louis congresswoman who helped secure federal money for the arch project. On this part of the walk, you will have great views of the Mississippi River and of the arch, which towers overhead.

➤Turn right and go up the fifty-four steps of the grand staircase to the memorial's park and plaza. Behind you to the east is East St. Louis, Illinois. In front of you is downtown St. Louis and lovely views of the Old Courthouse, with its large green dome, and the Old Cathedral, with its spire and cross. About halfway up the stairs you will find a plaque that marks the high-water mark of the 1993 flood.

➤Walk to your left and toward the south leg of the arch. Follow the sidewalk that takes you toward the Basilica of Saint Louis, King of France, known as the Old Cathedral.

This Greek Revival church sits on the spot Laclède had designated as the settlement's church block. Finished in 1834, it was once the mother church for more than half the Roman Catholics living in the United States. In the 1950s, when the city turned its attention to the Jefferson National Expansion Memorial, it included a facelift for the aging church. In 1961, Pope John XXIII made the church a minor basilica. The half-opened umbrella on display in the church is the symbol of its basilica status. Today the church is popular with worshippers and tourists.

As you step inside, note the French inscription above the portico, a reminder that St. Louis once was a French-speaking community. The large windows give the interior a surprisingly light, almost stark feel. The painting to the right of St. Louis praying was a gift from King Louis XVIII.

➤As you leave the church, turn to your right toward the sidewalk that travels along the basilica's west wall. Here you will find the entrance to the church's museum. Continue along this sidewalk to the spot where Market Street meets Memorial Drive.

➤At Market, turn left and cross Memorial Drive.

➤When you have crossed the interstates, turn right and walk in front of the gardens on the east side of the Old Courthouse. From this spot you will have wonderful views of both the courthouse and the arch. The courthouse has a split architectural personality. Begun in the Greek Revival style, it was finished in the Italian Renaissance style, which had become more popular. When the Civil Courts Building was completed in 1930, the Old Courthouse was retired. The people of St. Louis deeded the building and land to the U.S. government for its inclusion in the national park.

➤At Chestnut Street, turn left and walk to Broadway.

➤At Broadway, turn left and walk along the west side of the Old Courthouse. You will find information about the courthouse on page 28 of Walk 1 and in Appendix B.

➤Continue down Broadway. Busch Stadium is ahead. After you cross Walnut Street, you will have a sidewalk view of the seats inside the stadium.

➤Continue on Broadway across the street from the stadium until you reach Spruce.

➤At Spruce, cross Broadway and head to your right toward Stadium Plaza, walking along the stadium's south side. Watch for traffic.

➤Follow the sidewalk around the stadium.

Named for the Anheuser-Busch Brewery—the stadium's major donor—the Cardinal's home field was dedicated May 12, 1966. Busch Stadium was built in the downtown area to lure fans back into the city's core. The plan worked. On game days—especially when the Cardinals's big rival, the Chicago Cubs, are in town—this area overflows with activity.

The stadium resembles Rome's Colosseum in size and appearance. Its architect, however, added a distinctive St. Louis touch by repeating the Gateway Arch design ninety-six times on the stadium's exterior.

Between gates 5 and 6 on Walnut Street, you will find the entrance to the St. Louis Cardinals Hall of Fame and a gift shop that carries innumerable objects with the Cardinals's logo. Contact the stadium about its tours.

As you walk along the stadium's west side, look for the Bowling Hall of Fame and Museum across the street from the stadium's northwest corner. This handicapped-accessible museum pays tribute to a popular sport, detailing its 5,000-year-old history and development. Visitors can even bowl on an old-fashioned alley, complete with pin setters.

➤Cross Walnut at the crosswalk by the Mark Twain Bank and continue on Stadium Plaza, which is also 7th Street. As you cross Market, look off to your right for another fine view of the arch.

➤Continue on 7th to Chestnut. You will pass the Morton D. May Amphitheater in the Keiner Plaza on your right. With its flowing water, benches, and open areas, this plaza is popular with children and office workers looking for an outdoor lunch spot.

➤Turn left at Chestnut and cross 7th. You will follow Chestnut to 10th Street.

The building located at 111 North 7th is the architecturally admired Wainwright Building. Architect Louis Sullivan designed the building in 1891 for the businessman Ellis Wainwright. Sullivan's first skyscraper, this architectural landmark uses a steel frame instead of masonry to support its height. Although this building changed the skyline

All aboard!

No tour of St. Louis's downtown is complete without a trip into Union Station. Here you can play all day, watch chocolate goo turn into fudge, shop 'til you drop in unique stores, and eat and drink your fill. This lively and historic spot, once the world's busiest rail terminal, is now a National Historic Landmark.

Designed by Theodore C. Link in a Richardsonian Romanesque style, the terminal cost $6.5 million to build and covered more than ten acres. When it opened on September 1, 1894, it was the largest rail terminal in the country with nineteen miles of track in its yards. More than 20,000 people came to its opening-night party.

With its turrets, limestone facade, and red roof, it resembles a medieval walled city. Its large clock tower—the symbol of St. Louis before the arch—soars above a building that stretches for two blocks. The Grand Hall, trimmed in gold leaf and decorated with stained glass windows, frescoes, elaborate light fixtures, and statuary, surely impressed the more than 100,000 travelers who passed under its 65-foot barrel-vault ceiling each day. Today the hall is an elegant hotel lobby.

After World War II, rail travel declined. The last train pulled out of Union Station on October 31, 1978.

Restored and refitted, the station reopened in August 1985. At a cost of $150 million, it was the largest adaptive re-use project in the United States. Today, this city within a city includes more than one hundred shops and restaurants, the Hyatt Regency Hotel, a lake with paddle boats, and a ferris wheel and carousel.

Those interested in the station's history can enjoy an award-winning collection of letters, memorabilia, and exhibits displayed throughout the station area. A self-guided walking tour shares a great deal about this once-vital terminal.

of interest

The Grand Tour

Spend a day walking downtown St. Louis. If you combine Walks 1 through 3, you can cover seven miles in the city's heart. The walk will take about four hours, but add at least another four hours to visit the arch, the Old Courthouse, Union Station, and any other building or area that attracts your attention. You will also need to take time to eat, and with an array of good restaurants, you certainly will not go hungry or thirsty. Union Station and the St. Louis Centre should also satisfy any shopper.

Start at the MetroLink stop in Laclede's Landing and follow the directions for Walk 2, which start on page 31.

After Walk 2, cross Washington Street and enter the Jefferson National Memorial Park, either from the upper level of the parking garage or at the sidewalk at Washington and Memorial Drive.

Follow the directions for Walk 1, which begin on page 19. At the end of Walk 1, you will once again be at the corner of Washington and Memorial Drive.

Turn left on Memorial and walk toward the Old Cathedral. The river will be on your left and the Old Courthouse will be on your right.

Cross Memorial Drive at Walnut Street.

Follow Walnut Street to Broadway.

Turn left on Broadway and head toward Busch Stadium. Turn to page 47 of Walk 3 and pick up the directions as they guide you past the stadium and on to Union Station.

After you have walked to the 20th Street entrance of Union Station, go out the 20th Street door. Turn right and go to the corner, which is 20th and Market. Walk 3 starts at this corner. Go to page 40 and the start of Walk 3.

Follow the Walk 3 directions until they return you to the Laclede's Landing MetroLink stop.

of American cities, Sullivan died poor and forgotten. His pupil Frank Lloyd Wright captured the architectural spotlight.

➤At 10th Street, turn left and walk one block to Market.

➤Cross Market, then turn to your right and cross 10th.

➤Continue on Market to 18th Street.

➤Cross 18th and turn to your left. Go into Union Station through its 18th Street entrance.

➤Walk through the station's lower level to the 20th Street entrance. When you exit this door, turn right and go to the corner, where this walk ends. As you walk through the station, you will pass the entrance into the Hyatt Hotel on your right. Be sure to go up the stairs and admire the Grand Hall and the stained glass windows. Unless you are pressed for time, do not leave Union Station without exploring this wonderful area.

walk 4
Park Tour

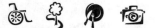

General location: Forest Park is due west of downtown near the city's western edge.

Special attractions: Magnificent and expansive city park, museums, zoo, pastoral setting, boating and fishing.

Difficulty rating: Hike-bike path is paved and level; city sidewalks occasionally uneven.

Distance: 4 miles.

Estimated time: 2 hours.

Services: Restrooms, drinking fountains, restaurants.

Restrictions: Dogs must be leashed. Group picnicking only in designated areas. The first three-quarters of the path follows the park's hike-bike path and is fully accessible to the handicapped. However, curbing, a few stairs, and an occasional absence of sidewalk in the final leg of the trail make the path inaccessible between the St. Louis Art Museum and the Jefferson Memorial Building. People in wheelchairs or those pushing strollers can catch the Shuttle Bug at the art museum and ride back to the start point.

For more information: Contact the St. Louis Convention and Visitors Commission or the Forest Park office.

Getting started: This walk starts in front of the Jefferson Memorial Building, which is at the intersection of Lindell Boulevard and DeBaliviere Avenue. To get to the memorial, take Interstate 64/40 to either the Kingshighway Boulevard or Skinker Boulevard exits and go north to Lindell Boulevard. Turn on Lindell so that you are heading toward the park. The Jefferson Memorial Building is about halfway between Skinker and Kingshighway. Parking is available near the building.

Public transportation: The MetroLink stop for Forest Park is on DeBaliviere and just one block from the start point.

Overview: With more than thirteen hundred acres, this park is larger than New York's Central Park. Dedicated in 1876, the park took its name from the natural forest that once covered this area.

Named one of the top ten urban parks in the country, Forest Park welcomes thousands of people each day, and no wonder. Within this large, grassy rectangle you will find the St. Louis Art Museum; the Missouri History Museum in the imposing Jefferson Memorial Building; St. Louis Science Center and Planetarium; the Jewel Box with its seasonal horticulture displays; the Muny, the city's outdoor concert arena; the zoo; the World's Fair Pavilion; and the Steinberg Skating Rink. Dozens of tennis courts and sports fields, several lakes, picnic grounds, hiking and biking trails, bridle paths, and boating and fishing opportunities round out the outdoor options.

Forest Park Tour

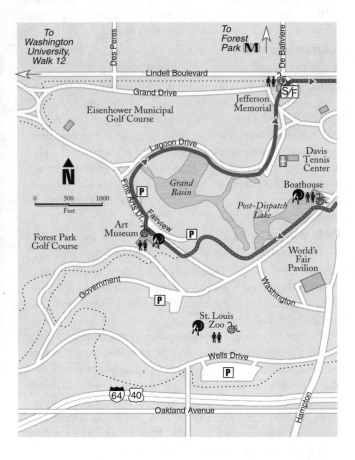

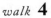

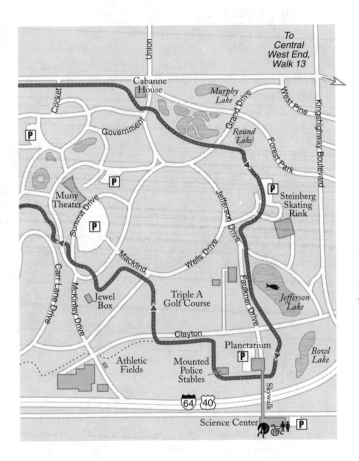

of interest

Meet me at the fair

In 1904, the western half of Forest Park was the site for part of the St. Louis World's Fair, which many state historians consider a defining moment in Missouri history. During its seven months, the fair welcomed more than 20 million visitors from around the world and put the city on the world stage.

Officially known as the Louisiana Purchase Exposition, the fair commemorated the centennial of the actual transfer of land from France to the United States. This transfer represented the world's largest real estate deal: $15 million for 825,000 square miles, or 528 million acres. As a cost and size comparison, the fourteen hundred acres purchased for Forest Park cost $800,000 in 1874.

Today, when electric lights, Disney World, and mass communication and transportation are mundane rather than magical, it is hard to imagine the enchantment and wonder the fair inspired. As fair organizers intended, most of the structures, landscaping, and amusements were removed once the fair was over. Only two of the exposition palaces were meant to be permanent. The rest were made of staff—a mixture of plaster of Paris and fibers—spread over temporary wooden Frames and were torn down. You must use your imagination to re-create the fair's glory.

You can no longer walk the fairgrounds; golf courses sit on the sites of many exhibits. But this walk and part of Walk 12 will take you through a large portion of the fair's areas and tell you what you would have seen were you strolling here between May and November in 1904.

Until 2001, the Missouri History Museum will feature "Meet Me at the Fair: Memory, History and the 1904 World's Fair." Artifacts, photos, recorded recollections, and extensive historical detail will help you experience this magnificent exposition. When the exhibit closes, the museum will continue to be the greatest repository of fair memorabilia.

The walk

This walk starts in the front of the Jefferson Memorial Building, which stands at the former main gate to the World's Fair. Dedicated in 1913, the building was funded through fair profits and has always been home to the Missouri Historical Society. Before or after this walk, visit the Missouri History Museum exhibits and its interesting gift shop.

In 1904, the Pike—the fair's exciting mile-and-a-half-long amusement strip—would have been off to your right and just on the other side of Lindell Boulevard. Described as "an enchanted thoroughfare of adventure and light-hearted revelry," the Pike gave visitors a taste of exotic food and drink, a peek at war re-enactments and infant incubators with live babies, and exhibits such as the Tyrolean Alps, the Irish village, Asia, Cairo, and water chutes and magic whirlpools.

Many locals wanted the Pike and its merrymaking to continue after the fair closed. But opposition, especially from nearby Washington University, was too strong. By the 1930s, an upscale residential area obliterated any signs of this fun-filled strip.

➤As you face the grand fountain, turn to your left and follow the sidewalk.

➤Cross DeBaliviere and pick up the hike-bike trail on the other side. This trail goes around the park, covers about seven miles, and is enjoyed by hikers, bikers, and in-line skaters. The path can get crowded, so watch for fast-moving travelers.

➤Cross Cricket Drive and continue on the path, which soon will veer away from Lindell and go deep into the park.

➤At the intersection of Grand and Government drives, you will cross the multilane street and its median strip and pick up the hike-bike path on the other side.

On either side you will see signs of the park's canal system and lagoons and aerated ponds, or fish hatchery lakes; the lagoons were once managed by the U.S. Bureau of Fisheries. About five feet deep, these watering holes are now enjoyed by ducks and geese.

➤When you come upon Grand Drive again, obey the yield sign and watch for traffic before picking up the path on the other side. On your left you will see Round Lake, which spouts a ninety-foot spray in warm weather. As you enter an area accessible only to walkers and bikers, you leave behind the park's bustle and traffic.

➤The parking for the Steinberg Skating Rink will come up on your left. A gift from Mark C. Steinberg Charitable Trust, the rink opened in 1957 and took its inspiration from the skating pond in New York's Central Park.

➤Cross the road and continue on the bike path, which now parallels Wells Drive.

➤At the intersection of Jefferson and Wells drives, follow the path as it curves and heads toward Jefferson Lake. You will soon pass the path's one-mile marker and will have a better view of the skating rink.

➤Cross Jefferson and watch for traffic. You are now walking parallel to Faulkner Drive. The hike-bike trail picks up on the other side of Jefferson and takes you along Jefferson Lake. The sign notes that this fishing lake is home to largemouth bass, channel cat, crappie, and carp. The buildings you see on the other side of the lake are the city's hospital complex: Barnes-Jewish Hospital and Children's Hospital. With the lake and limited traffic, the park now feels more remote and pastoral.

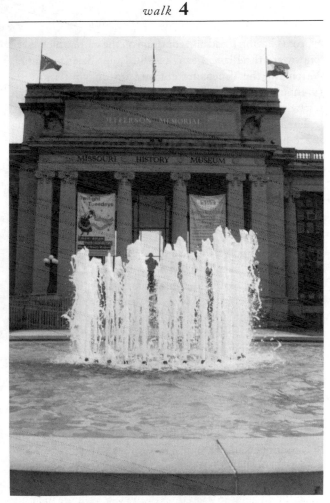

The Missouri History Museum, housed in the Jefferson Memorial, offers extensive and imaginative displays of St. Louis history.

➤Cross Clayton Road and continue on the path, which takes you toward the Planetarium and St. Louis Science Center. Watch for the dinosaurs coming up on your right—a Tyrannosaurus rex and a triceratops. The sign says you can touch them and take their pictures, but you must not feed them.

The Planetarium is on your right, and the main building of the Science Center is to your left, on the other side of Interstate 64/40. If you would like to visit the Science Center before continuing on this walk, take the path that comes up on your left. It leads to the skywalk that goes over the highway and connects to the center. While in the skywalk, use one of the radar guns to clock the speed of the traffic as it whizzes by.

The St. Louis Science Center, billed as "the playground for your mind," brings you face-to-face with two life-size animatronic dinosaurs that move and roar. You can journey through mines, a brick sewer, and a modern utility tunnel; peer inside an actual Gemini space capsule; or try your hand at surgery! The museum is fully accessible and offers strollers, telecommunication devices for the deaf, braille visitor guides, and assistive listening devices. It also has a self-service restaurant and a gift shop offering educational toys and games, books, and fossils.

➤Just past the Planetarium are the stables for the mounted police. You may see officers on horseback during your walk. In front of you and to your left are playing fields.

➤The hike-bike path goes by the stables and then parallels the playing fields. In the summer, this tree-lined path offers welcome shade.

➤Follow the path as it turns left and parallels Clayton Road. You will soon seen the two-mile marker, and when you do, look across the street and locate where the hike-bike path heads off into the golf course.

➤Carefully cross the street and continue on this leg of the hike-bike path. The other leg of the trail continues west along Clayton Road.

➤Follow the path through the golf course. This portion of the trail has white fencing on either side.

➤After you leave the fencing, the hike-bike path curves, and you will come upon a yield sign at Wells Drive.

➤Cross Wells and continue on the hike-bike trail. In the summer, a drinking fountain off to your right, across the street, and by the softball field may offer refreshment.

➤Wells turns into Macklind Drive. On your left, as you walk along Macklind, you will see what appear to be Grecian ruins. You are entering the Jewel Box area, with its rose garden, benches, lily pond, and an upright sundial that remembers the veterans of the Korean War. An unconventional greenhouse, the Jewel Box was designed to withstand Midwest hailstorms. Built in 1936, it is open daily and offers seasonal floral displays.

➤Follow the hike-bike path across the street. Union Drive is not as busy as some park thoroughfares, but watch for traffic.

➤Cross Summit Drive and continue on the bike path with McKinley Drive running parallel on your left.

➤Cross McKinley. Watch for traffic in this busier area. The building coming up on your right is the Muny, a 12,000-seat outdoor theater. The oldest and largest of this country's outdoor theaters, its stage is half the length of a football field; its first show opened in 1919. Today its summer season includes musicals, Broadway shows, light opera, and dance.

After you cross McKinley and approach Concourse Drive, the hike-bike trail briefly becomes the actual sidewalk. Look

Fair facts

➤The fair covered 1,270 acres and cost $50 million.

➤George Kessler, creator of Kansas City's park system, was its chief landscape architect.

➤It was the first time electric lights lit up the outdoors.

➤About 50 countries and 45 states and territories were represented.

➤Indoor exhibits covered 5 million square feet of space; outdoor exhibits covered 6 million.

➤The ice cream cone, iced tea, and hot dogs are said to have originated at the fair.

➤The fair boasted the world's largest pipe organ and cascading fountains.

➤Scott Joplin played on the amusement strip known as the Pike and wrote "The Cascades" for the fair.

➤The song "Meet Me in St. Louis," was written for the Pike.

➤Each car of the 264-foot-high Observation Wheel, or ferris wheel, was the size of a trolley car and could seat forty-five people.

➤Ota Benga, an African pygmy who was captured by slave hunters, was put on display at the fair.

➤Other native peoples from the Philippines, Japan, and North America agreed to live at the fair temporarily as animated anthropological exhibits.

➤The fair's opening day, April 30, 1904, was a state and city holiday.

➤The fair made a profit, unlike most subsequent world fairs.

for the hike-bike path coming up on your right and take it. This part of the path will wind through a wooded area and over some bridges before coming out near the park's boathouse and Post-Dispatch Lake. You are now entering the part of Forest Park that was the site of the 1904 World's Fair; the rest of this walk will be on former fairgrounds.

➤Take the path across Government Drive and walk toward the Boathouse Cafe and the lake. Here you will find restrooms and a drinking fountain. Between April and October, the Boathouse Cafe serves lunch and dinner on its veranda overlooking the lake. On a summer evening, when the water catches the cafe's lights, this spot can be quite romantic.

Post-Dispatch Lake sits where exhibit halls for Mines and Metallurgy, and Liberal Arts stood during the fair. From this lake, you can rent a boat and sail into what remains of the fair's Grand Basin and look up at Art Hill and the St. Louis Art Museum.

➤When you are ready to leave the boathouse area, return to Government, turn right, and continue on the hike-bike path. The lake is to your right and off to your left and atop a hill is the World's Fair Pavilion, which gives its visitors a commanding view of Forest Park and the fairgrounds. This large building with its water spray commemorates the fair and was built on the site of the fair's Missouri Building. The state's exhibition hall was to be one of the fair's two permanent buildings, but it burned just before the fair closed.

➤Coming up on your left, as you approach the stop sign intersection at Washington and Government Drives, you will see the zoo entrance. Walk 5 on page 68 will walk you through the zoo, if you would like to explore it now. If you want to catch the Shuttle Bug, its stop is directly across from the zoo on Government Drive.

of interest

The St. Louis Art Museum

Built as the Palace of Art for the World's Fair, this facility was the first art museum west of the Mississippi River. Its Roman Revival design is the work of Cass Gilbert, who designed the U.S. Supreme Court Building.

Since 1907, public taxes have supported the art museum—the first American art museum to be municipally supported. It remains the only major U.S. art museum that still is "free to all," and it welcomes more than half a million visitors each year.

The museum houses an extensive collection representing ancient to contemporary art. However, its German Expressionist paintings and pre-Columbian collection rank among the world's best. The museum also has a gift shop and a popular restaurant. The Museum Cafe overlooks a courtyard with sculptures and a waterfall and offers a changing lunch menu and a popular Sunday brunch.

➤Whereas Washington Drive ends at the zoo, your hike-bike path curves off to your right. If you did not take a moment to refresh yourself at the boathouse, catch the bench that overlooks the lake.

➤Coming up on your right is the parking lot for the art museum. Soon you will see the museum, the only original fair building that still stands today.

Coming up on your right is the statue *Apotheosis of Saint Louis*, which depicts the patron saint of the city, who also reigned as King Louis IX of France in the thirteenth century. He is armored and ready to ride his steed into battle, his sword upended so that its handle forms a cross.

Originally made of staff sculpted over wood, the figure stood at the fair's main entrance on Lindell Boulevard. It was recast in bronze and placed above the Grand Basin in 1906. From here, rider and horse look out over Art Hill as it slopes toward the Grand Basin. In the winter, this hill offers the city's best sledding.

You now stand at one of the fair's most visually beautiful spots. The Grand Basin, with its cascading water and first-ever outdoor lighting, was the fair's dramatic centerpiece. More than ninety thousand gallons of water per minute poured down the terraces and into the basin; and at night, twenty thousand lights made the water sparkle. Just below this spot stood Festival Hall, with a 3,500-seat auditorium that housed the world's largest pipe organ. Its dome was said to be larger than St. Peter's in Rome.

➤When you reach Fine Arts Drive in front of the art museum, you will leave the hike-bike path. From here to the walk's end, you will walk along the park's less accessible sidewalks. Watch your footing as you may encounter some uneven surfaces, a few steps, and occasional curbing. Those pushing strollers or wheelchairs may want to catch the Shuttle Bug in front of the museum and ride back to the Jefferson Memorial Building.

➤If you are walking, cross Fine Arts Drive and walk along the front of the museum. You will get a better view of the building and also an expansive view of the park. Traffic may be heavy, so cross carefully.

➤When the sidewalk ends, recross the street and angle into Fairview Drive, walking carefully in the parking area between the parked cars. About four car lengths in, you will see where the sidewalk picks up again.

➤Take the sidewalk, which includes a few stairs, and resume your walk. The golf course to your left sits where the fair's Walled City of Jerusalem stood. This replica of the ancient holy city represented the many cultures and religions found within its walls and included Christ's birthplace, the Mosque of Omar and the Wailing Wall.

➤At the intersection accented with grass, flowers, and a statue of Edward Bates—U.S. attorney general under Lincoln—follow the sidewalk to the right. You are now walking along Lagoon Drive, which cuts through the golf course. Off to your right you will catch a different view of the Grand Basin and the front of the museum.

From this vantage point, fair goers could take in the beauty of the elaborately lighted water area and Festival Hall. Though less dramatic today, this spot still offers a beautiful view and a place to imagine the grandeur of the 1904 World's Fair. Grab a bench and enjoy the sights.

➤After you cross a little curved street, you will be heading toward the tennis courts and the Dwight Davis Tennis Center, named for the tennis player and parks commissioner who also established the Davis Cup. The courts will come up on your right.

➤You will leave the sidewalk and walk along the shoulder of Lagoon Drive. The walking area is wide at this point, but watch for traffic.

➤When you approach a driveway that says, "Do Not Enter," cross the street carefully, watching for traffic. Follow the combination of grass-and-dirt path and sidewalks that clearly angle you back to the Jefferson Memorial Building and the start of this walk.

of interest

Catch the Bug

If you get tired or simply want an enjoyable ride, hop the Shuttle Bug. You can ride all day for a buck and get on and off as you please. From the MetroLink's Forest Park station on DeBaliviere, this small, wheelchair-accessible red bus with black spots stops within Forest Park at the Missouri History Museum, the St. Louis Art Museum, the zoo, the Muny, the Jewel Box, and the St. Louis Science Center. It then leaves the park and travels east to the MetroLink's Central West End station by the hospital complex. From there it heads north to the shopping and dining area in the Central West End, and then on to the cathedral before looping back to the MetroLink's Forest Park stop.

If you want to walk through the art and history museums, science center, and the zoo, you may want to rest your feet by including a few Shuttle Bug connections in your walk.

If you have some energy after your Forest Park excursion, you can take the bug to the start of Walk 13. Pick up the Shuttle Bug outside the Jefferson Memorial Building and ride to the Central West End MetroLink stop and Walk 13, which starts on page 138.

walk 5

St. Louis Zoo

General location: In Forest Park, directly west of downtown.

Special attractions: World-famous zoo with more than 3,600 animals in naturalistic settings, plus the original, walk-through birdcage from the 1904 World's Fair.

Difficulty rating: Easy, completely flat, and on paved surfaces.

Distance: 1.5 miles.

Estimated time: 1 hour.

Services: Restaurants, souvenir and gift shops, several restrooms on the grounds, stroller and wheelchair rentals.

Restrictions: No pets, bicycles, skateboards, Rollerblades, or loud radios. Visitors may not feed the animals.

For more information: Contact the St. Louis Zoological Park.

Getting started: The zoo is in the south-central part of Forest Park. Interstate 64 runs directly along the park's southern border. From I-64, take the Hampton Avenue Museums-Zoo exit and follow the signs for the zoo. From Interstate 44, take the Hampton Avenue exit. Follow Hampton north one mile to the zoo. The walk starts from the zoo's Living World entrance just off Government Drive and the north parking lot. You can park for free along the street or for a small fee in the zoo lot.

Public transportation: Two Bi-State Transit buses—52 and 90—stop at the zoo. Bus 52 starts at the downtown terminal at Broadway and Locust Street. Bus 90, which runs on the western side of the city, cuts through Forest Park and stops at two of the zoo's three entrances. You can also take the MetroLink to the Forest Park stop and catch the Shuttle Bug. This small, red with black dots stops about every fifteen minutes at the MetroLink station and will let you off near The Living World entrance. Contact Bi-State Transit to confirm times, routes and fares.

Overview: By law and tradition, the St. Louis Zoo is free. In 1916, St. Louisans voted two-to-one to support the zoo through their taxes and to keep it "forever free to the usage of the inhabitants." They were the first citizens in the world to vote to support their local zoo. Modest fees for the Children's Zoo, Sea Lion Show, the Zooline Railroad, and tram system, food and souvenir sales, plus the zoo's well-known work with endangered species—including successful breeding programs—now help support the facility.

In the late 1800s, the city had a makeshift zoo. When the Smithsonian brought its giant flight cage to the 1904 World's Fair, people considered building a zoo around it. But it was not until 1913 that the city's Municipal Assembly set aside seventy-seven acres within Forest Park to house the city's growing collection of animals.

St. Louis Zoo

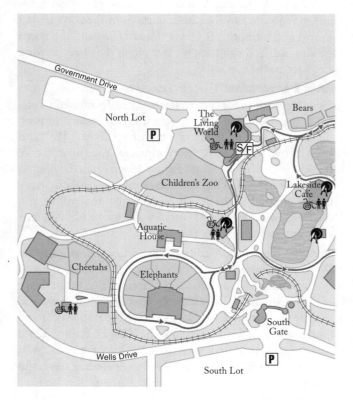

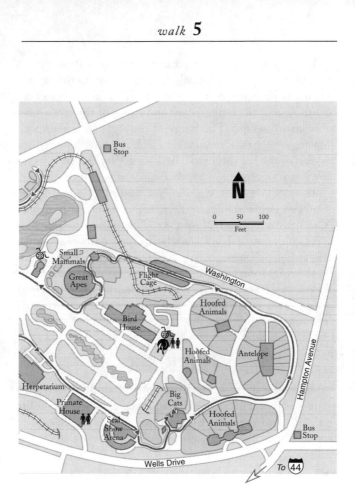

Once considered the country's finest zoo, it pioneered the practice of placing animals in open enclosures that mimic the natural environment. Today the St. Louis Zoo still remains among the nation's best and is one of the city's most popular attractions. The Jungle of the Apes with glass-wall viewing, the newly remodeled children's zoo, an open-air exhibit of the big cats, and The Living World—an interactive learning center—draw thousands of visitors each year.

In good weather, the Zooline Railroad—one of the country's larger miniature railroads—operates from mid-March through mid-November. The train is wheelchair accessible and offers a round-trip tour of the zoo with reboarding privileges.

With its paved and level pathways, natural animal settings, waterfalls, ponds, and well-tended and spacious grounds, the zoo offers an ideal walk for everyone, regardless of age or ability.

The walk

This walk starts in The Living World. Built in 1989, this state-of-the-art educational center teaches people about life on earth and the ways in which nature works. Be sure to spend some time in the center either before or after your walk.

➤Turn to your right after leaving The Living World and go down the ramp.

➤Turn left at the bottom of the ramp. You are heading toward the elephants. On your right is the Children's Zoo.

To your left, you will see a small lake, home to swans and ducks. After you cross the Zooline tracks, you will see a picnic pavilion, a snack bar, and accessible restrooms.

➤At the first major intersection, take the road going off to your right. This large outside enclosure is home to Asian elephants. Follow the path to the right around this enclosure, which is ringed with benches. The first building on your right is the Aquatic House; inside you will find penguins and a school of piranhas.

Coming up on your right, on the other side of the tracks, is the Cheetah Survival Center. To the right and across the tracks are accessible restrooms.

➤Continue your circle around the open-air pens until you reach the entrance to the Elephant House. Inside you will find a species of wild pig that comes from the Togian Isles. As you complete your circle, you will come to a path on your right that leads to the zoo's south gate. A railroad station is just beyond. Take this path to your right if you need information, a TDD phone, gift shop, or family restrooms.

➤Your path around the Elephant House ends where you first entered this area. Turn right and go down the walkway. Where several paths intersect, you will walk past the wooden marker and follow the path that curves right. The lake is in front of you and will be on your left as you head down the path. Look for the many varieties of waterfowl that splash here.

➤Follow the arrows that point toward the big cats, the primates, herpetarium, and the sea lion show. The lake will be behind you as you head toward these exhibits.

The Herpetarium, with its name marked above the door, appears first. Images of its inhabitants have been incorporated into the building design. Next comes the Primate House. Its wheelchair-accessible entrance is on the west side. Both of these buildings were built in the 1920s and remodeled in the 1970s. Next come the Seal Show Arena and then Big Cat Country, which is obvious from the high meshing that covers the cat pits.

➤Follow the path as it curves around and above the cat exhibit. The black iron fence will be on your left as you curve around.

➤Circle the cat area and return to the spot where you entered. The path will take you past the hoofed animal exhibits with zebras, antelope, and camels. Watch for okapis, and, on your left, emus and kangaroos. The entrance to the Antelope House will come up on your left. You may enter the house and exit from the opposite end. If the weather is nice, however, you may want to follow the path around the Antelope House and view the animals in their outdoor pens.

➤Continue on the path as it circles the hoofed animal exhibits and then follow the signs for the 1904 Flight Cage. A slightly inclined path with a brick wall and railings will take you to the cage, one of only two structures surviving from the 1904 fair.

➤Enter the birdcage. Part of the U.S. exhibit and sponsored by the Smithsonian Institution at the 1904 fair, the cage was made 50 feet high, 84 feet wide and 228 feet long. It appears today much as it did in 1904. When the fair ended, the Smithsonian sold the cage to the city for $6,000. It is still one of the world's largest free-flight aviaries and is home to numerous birds. A wooden walkway will take you past the flamingo and lush vegetation and over the pools.

➤When you come out the other end, you will cross the railroad tracks and take the first path heading off to your left toward the Jungle of the Apes. You will see large rocks and a waterfall. An incline ramp will take you along the waterfall and the animals' outdoor area. The building's entrance is at the top of the incline. The splashing sound of water and the earthy smell of vegetation and primates gives a pleasant jungle feel as the path winds you gently upward around the rocks and the animals. When you leave

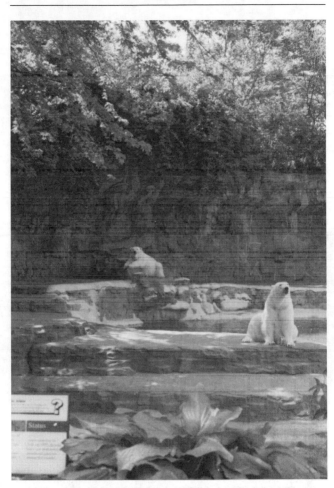

The bear pits, modeled after the bluffs along the Mississippi River, were among the first exhibits designed for the St. Louis Zoo.

the building, be sure to check the outdoor exhibits to see if any gorillas or orangutans are lounging outdoors.

➤Turn to your right when you leave the primates and walk between the wood pylons into a picnic grove. The Lakeside Cafe is the large hexagonal building to your right. The seal pond is directly in front of you.

➤Walk toward the seals and then turn right and take the path past the seals and toward the Lakeside Cafe.

➤Follow the roadway that curves along and then past the Lakeside Cafe. A large duck pond is on your right.

➤After you cross the railroad tracks, turn right on the path that goes toward the rocks and waterfalls of the bear pits. Here you will find several bear species: polar, speckled, grizzly, and American black. These bear pits were completed in 1919 and were designed to resemble the bluffs along the Mississippi River. They became a popular model for other zoos.

➤Walk to the end of the bear exhibits and then double back. In the heat of a St. Louis summer, this shaded path and sounds of splashing water are especially refreshing.

➤Head back toward The Living World and the end of your walk.

If you want to take the Shuttle Bug to other park attractions, the Cathedral Basilica of St. Louis, or the Central West End, you can catch it outside the Living World Entrance and to your right. You can also take this little bus to the start of Walks 4 and 13 or to the MetroLink stations for Forest Park and the Central West End. Both of these station stops are featured in Walk 15.

walk 6

Missouri Botanical Garden

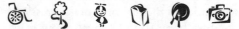

General location: South-central area of the city, just west of the Anheuser-Busch Brewery.

Special attractions: Beautifully maintained gardens on seventy-nine acres, including the fourteen-acre Japanese Garden, the smaller English and Chinese gardens, the Climatron conservatory, and Tower Grove House.

Difficulty rating: Easy, flat, all on paved paths.

Distance: 2 miles.

Estimated time: 1 hour.

Services: Several restrooms, restaurant, gift shop, tram, tours with garden guides. Wheelchairs and assistive listening devices available.

Restrictions: No pets, picnicking, coolers, or lawn furniture in the garden. Shirts and shoes required; collecting live plants, flowers, or fruits forbidden.

For more information: Contact the Missouri Botanical Garden.

Getting started: The Missouri Botanical Garden is bordered by Tower Grove Avenue to the east, Alfred Avenue to the west, Magnolia Avenue to the south, and Shaw Boulevard to the north. Its entrance is off Shaw. From Interstate 44 or Interstate 64/40, take the Kingshighway Exit south to Vandeventer. Turn left onto Vandeventer and go to Shaw. Turn right on Shaw and proceed to the garden's entrance. Park for free in the large lots on either side of the entrance.

Public transportation: Bi-State Transit Bus 99 starts at the main bus terminal at Broadway and Locust and stops at the garden. Contact Bi-State Transit to confirm times and other bus routes.

Overview: Henry Shaw created the Missouri Botanical Garden—the first such garden in the nation—on the grassland surrounding his country home Tower Grove. Shaw made his fortune selling hardware to settlers heading west and retired at the ripe young age of forty. After traveling abroad for several years, he returned to St. Louis and focused his attentions on this garden and Tower Grove Park, a few blocks away. The many notable gardens in his native England inspired him to create public gardens for the people of St. Louis. He opened this garden in 1859.

In addition to being a delightful place to stroll, the Missouri Botanical Garden also houses a major botanical library and the William T. Kemper Center for Home Gardening. It is also a world leader in botanical and environmental research, with an emphasis on the study of rain forests and the planet's overall environmental quality.

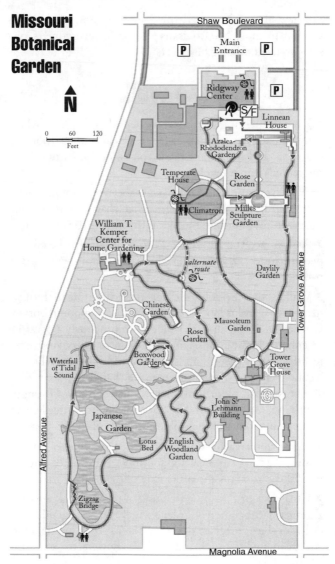

Missouri Botanical Garden

Shaw Boulevard

Main Entrance

P   P   P

Ridgway Center

S/F   Linnean House

Azalea-Rhododendron Garden

Temperate House

Rose Garden

Climatron

Mille's Sculpture Garden

William T. Kemper Center for Home Gardening

alternate route

Daylily Garden

Chinese Garden

Rose Garden

Mausoleum Garden

Tower Grove House

Boxwood Garden

Waterfall of Tidal Sound

Japanese Garden

Lotus Bed

John S. Lehmann Building

Zigzag Bridge

English Woodland Garden

Tower Grove Avenue

Alfred Avenue

Magnolia Avenue

N

0   60   120
Feet

Shaw always intended this garden—known as Shaw's Garden to most St. Louisans—to be for everyone. Consider yourself among his guests.

The walk

➤From the parking lot, walk into the Ridgway Center where you will pay your admission fee. You will find restrooms, a gift shop, and restaurant here. You enter the garden from the center's upper level.

➤When you enter the garden, walk ahead toward the Latzer Fountain. If you are pushing a wheelchair or stroller, you can reach the fountain by taking the incline to your right.

➤As you face the fountain, go to your left. In the spring, purple pansies, azaleas, and yellow snapdragons will line the path.

➤Walk across Spoehrer Plaza toward Linnean House, named for Carolus Linnaeus, the founder of modern botany. Opened in 1882, it is the oldest, continuously operating greenhouse in the country and one of the few surviving nineteenth-century greenhouses in the world. The camellia collection has been displayed for more than a hundred years and bursts into bloom in January and February. Throughout the year, you will find a variety of plants. Enter by way of the stairs or by the accessible entrance off the brick patio.

➤Leave this area by walking between the bushes and go toward the carp waterfall and fountain. You are heading toward the garden on the other side of the bridge.

➤Cross the bridge or enter under the pergola into the Zimmerman Scented Garden, which was designed especially for the blind. The flower bed signs are in braille. Here you are invited to touch and smell the flowers, to "know the beauty that one can and cannot see," and to listen to the bells or to make them ring.

➤Continue on the path, which passes through hosta, coral bells, and the variegated goatweed. This path parallels Tower Grove Avenue, which is on the other side of the wall to your left. To your right, within the white fence, is the rose garden, which you will walk through later.

➤At the reflecting pond you can see the Climatron off to your right. The Climatron, home to plants from the rain forests as well as dry upland areas, was the first of its kind when it opened in 1960. You will walk through the geodesic dome and get a closer look at the sculptures toward the end of this walk.

➤You will pass through the iris beds as you walk straight ahead toward Tower Grove House and the Victorian Garden. In the spring, these iris beds are showy in deep purple and lavender, as well as flame yellow and orange.

➤The Jenkins Daylily Garden appears next and is most spectacular in the early summer. A huge towering pin oak comes up on your left, just past a large holly. The sculpture, *Victory of Science Over Ignorance*, was a gift from Shaw.

➤Continue to follow the signs for Tower Grove House, the Victorian Garden, the maze, and the Japanese Garden. Tower Grove is the white structure with dark green trim. This Italianate style country house was designed by George I. Barnett—Shaw's favorite architect—and was completed in 1849. This restored house includes many of Shaw's furnishings. Tours are available.

➤Keeping to the left, walk around Tower Grove. You will see a statue of Juno surrounded by a bed of annual flowers.

➤Walk into the herb garden, which is fenced with ornate, black wrought-iron. Walk toward the herb garden exit, which is at the opposite end. Be sure to take time to enjoy the herbs and to read the signs that tell you what is growing here.

➤As you exit the herb garden, take the path to the right. You will curve past the swamp white oak, and the *Fountain Angel* will be on your right. This sculpture originally stood at the 1904 World's Fair.

➤Follow the path as it curves to the left. You are heading toward the English Garden. To your left is the John S. Lehmann Building. A huge praying mantis on its roof makes it impossible to miss. This is the library, and it is not open to the public. Made of bronze overlaid on stainless steel, the Mantis honors an insect beneficial to gardeners. *Two Piece Reclining Figure No. 2*, by Henry Moore, is near the path on your left.

➤Enter the English Garden. On a hot summer day, this shady area with dappled sunlight is a delicious retreat. You will follow a maze-like path that loops around and through the various plantings.

➤Where the road forks, you will curve to the right. Do not leave the garden. Depending on the season, your senses will be bombarded by a variety of colors and textures. You will see other narrower paths cutting away and into the garden. Explore these if you wish, but come back to the paved path. Enjoy the ponds and bog garden with its algae, ferns, iris, and columbine.

➤Go to your left when you leave this garden. You will pass between two ginkgo trees.

➤At the next intersection, go left and follow the signs to the Japanese Garden, Seiwa-en. In this fourteen-acre strolling garden, you will see a lake, waterfall, bridges, and the ornamental plantings associated with Japanese landscaping.

As soon as you enter this garden, you will feel a sense of openness and expanse. Instead of flowers, this garden emphasizes landscape structure—lawns, evergreens, manicured and sculpted trees, a lotus pad, and the dry gravel garden with raked patterns. In the spring, your eyes and nose will delight to the peony bushes bearing fragrant, heavy blossoms of pink or white.

➤Before you cross the carp bridge, spend a dime and buy some food for the colorful koi swimming in this area. At the slightest hint of food, they will open their huge mouths and churn up the water as they vie for your pellets.

The dry gravel garden continues, punctuated by weeping cherries, which bloom in the late spring. To your left you will find accessible restrooms and a water fountain.

➤Past the restrooms the path curves. You will have your choice of staying on the paved path or walking across the wooden zigzag bridge. It is said the devil cannot follow you across a zigzag path. If you take the wooden bridge, you will feel as though you are walking across the surface of the water. The zigzag bridge returns you to the paved pathway.

➤Continue down the path until you come to the Drum Bridge, or Taikobashi Bridge, which will take you to the Teahouse Island. The bridge offers a peaceful vantage point from which to view the gardens. Nakajima, the sacred tea house, is closed to public.

➤Return to the path and continue past the rushing stream. You will hear the sound of running water and soon will see the waterfall. Shortly after the falls, you will come upon a slight fork in the road.

➤Stay on the path. To your left is the William T. Kemper Center for Home Gardening. To your right is the lake.

➤At a major Y intersection, take the left arm of the Y.

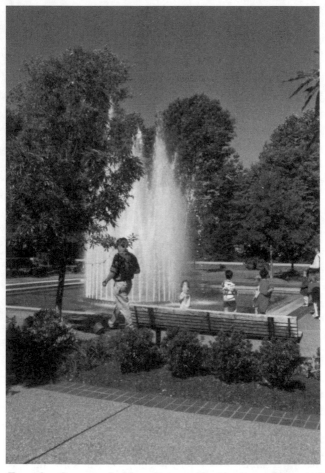

Fountains, flowers and wide walkways will add to your enjoyment of the Missouri Botanical Gardens.

➤At the tall, decorative brick wall, turn to your right. To your left is another entrance for the Home Gardening Center.

➤Enter the Boxwood Garden on your right, an elegant parterre in the shape of Henry Shaw's initials. You will find the "leaping waters" fountain and a gazebo. Explore the garden as you wish.

➤Return to the walkway that will take you back out the way you came in. As you leave you face the home garden area. If you wish, take a moment to explore the home gardening area and then return to this spot.

➤Turn to your right as you leave the Boxwood Garden.

➤A flagstone pathway will come up on your right. Take it and enter the Chinese Garden. Walk under the pagoda archway and into a tiny walled garden. Listen to the burbling water in this intimate space. If you wish, sit a moment in the pagoda and gaze into the reflection pool.

➤Cross the bridge and go through the moon gate.

➤Follow the flagstone pathway leading away from the garden and toward the Kemper Center.

➤Turn to the right and follow the main path. Do not take the path into the composting demonstration area.

➤Take the first right on a gray asphalt pathway and walk toward the Shapleigh Fountain with its circular spray of shooting water. Soon you will enter the Lehmann Rose Garden. The path that encircles the fountain offers two choices. To your right is the stairway entrance into the rose garden. To your left is a level path that leads away from the roses and toward the Climatron. If you are pushing a wheelchair, take the path to the left.

You may be able to carry a stroller up the eleven steps that are spaced out in the rose garden. If not, take the path toward the Climatron. If your party wishes to split up at this point, plan to meet at the dome; you will easily find each other outside the Climatron's main entrance on its west side.

➤Those taking the stairs soon will find themselves in the rose garden. As you face the Lehmann Rose Garden sign, take the path to your left. If the roses are blooming, you should be able to catch their perfume.

➤Follow the path toward the pavilion.

➤At the pavilion, go to the left around one side of the pavilion and take the first path that comes up on your left. You will find a water spray fountain and the path that leads to Tower Grove House.

➤At the T intersection, turn left and stay to your left as you follow the circular pathway.

➤Walk through the marble portals and enter the shaded mausoleum garden. The path will take you through the garden and along Shaw's mausoleum. Look for the tomb's stained glass windows.

➤When the path ends, turn left and walk toward the Climatron.

➤As you approach the geodesic dome, take the path that goes off to your left. The dome is now on your right, and you are taking the path around it.

➤At the intersection go right and follow the sign that directs you toward the Brookings Interpretive Center, Temperate House, and the Climatron. If you are rejoining your party, a spot by the fountain and benches would be an ideal place to meet.

➤Enter the Interpretive Center and go through the doors on the left, which take you into the Climatron. You will wind your way to the first exit that will come up on your left. In this rain forest, you will feel breezes, hear the ongoing sound of rushing water and waterfalls, and see many exotic trees: palms, a chocolate tree, pepper tree, orange tree, and avocado, to name a few.

➤When you reach the first exit on your left, go through the doors that say PUSH. To the left is Temperate House, which features species from the warm, dry regions. If you want to explore that garden, do so now and return to this spot.

➤After you exit the Climatron, take the path that goes off to your right and curves toward the ponds and fountain. The Climatron is now on your right.

➤Go left at your first chance and walk along the reflection pool, which is on your right. Here you will find the Milles Sculpture Garden—seven bronzes by Carl Milles in a pool with water lilies.

➤Where you see the three angles, curve to your left and follow the path that heads off to the left and toward the Linnean House. In the spring, this area is a sea of flowering bulbs.

➤Walk through the rose garden. If you wish to avoid the stairs, take the incline path to your left.

➤Walk around the fountain spray and head out of the garden.

➤Turn to your left and walk along the flower beds.

➤Then take a sharp left and follow the path to the dappled beds of rhododendron and azaleas.

➤At the statue of the family playing, make a right turn. In late May the red, purple, and white blossoms of rhododendron in bloom will greet you. Earlier in May the azaleas will be showy with blooms of white, orange, and pink.

➤Walk toward the tram station. From here you can see the entrance to the Ridgway Center and the end of this walk.

Be sure to visit the wonderful gift shop, which offers an array of garden-related items and an excellent selection of gardening books. The restaurant offers good food at reasonable prices, and in warm weather you can eat outdoors in view of the gardens.

walk 7

Park Tour

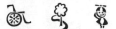

General location: Just south of the Missouri Botanical Garden in the south-central area of the city.

Special attractions: One of the world's few remaining Victorian parks, intriguing architectural details, fanciful gazebos, fountain and ponds, lush plantings.

Difficulty rating: Easy, completely accessible, perfect for joggers.

Distance: 2 miles.

Estimated time: 1 hour.

Services: Restrooms, picnic tables and shelters, grills, playgrounds, tennis courts, par course exercise circuit, and wading pool. Stupp Center for senior citizens open weekdays and by reservation evenings and weekends.

Park Tour

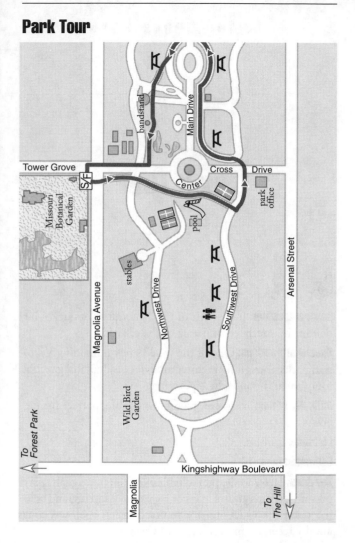

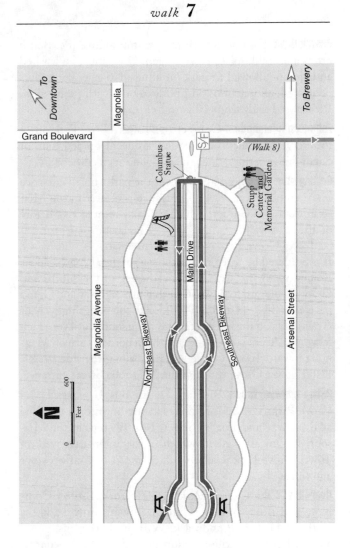

Restrictions: Do not disturb the plant or animal life. Boom boxes and loud noises discouraged. Dogs must be leashed and are not allowed in park buildings. No glass containers permitted, and alcohol on premises only with permission. Park closed daily from 10 p.m. to 5 a.m.

For more information: Contact the Tower Grove Park office to reserve park facilities, request a docent-guided tour, or obtain information about the park and its facilities.

Getting started: This walk starts at the park's north entrance on Magnolia Avenue. This entrance is closest to the Missouri Botanical Garden, which you may want to visit before or after this walk.

Tower Grove Park is south of Interstates 44 and 64/40. It is bordered by three major thoroughfares: Kingshighway Boulevard to the west, Arsenal Street to the south, and Grand Boulevard to the east. Both Kingshighway and Grand have exits off I-44 and I-64/40. Take the Kingshighway or Grand exits off the interstates and drive south until you reach Magnolia Avenue, the park's northern border. Turn on Magnolia toward Tower Grove and park along the side streets. Enter Tower Grove through the Magnolia Street entrance.

Public transportation: Bi-State Transit Bus 21 passes Tower Grove Park. The bus originates at the downtown terminal at Broadway and Locust Street. Bus 99 stops at the Missouri Botanical Garden, which is within an easy walk of Tower Grove Park. Call Bi-State Transit to confirm stops and times.

Overview: Like Central Park in New York, Boston Common, and Boston Public Garden, Tower Grove Park is a National Historic Landmark. With its faux ruins, grand gates, whimsical pavilions, statuary, and ponds, it is considered the best-preserved walking park in the nation and one of the few surviving Victorian parks in the world.

Henry Shaw, founder of the Missouri Botanical Garden, gave the land to the city in 1868 for the express purpose of creating a public park for strolling and concerts. He named it after his home, which is located nearby in the botanical garden.

When Shaw bought the land, it was virtually a treeless prairie. Today, this urban forest of 289 acres has more than eight thousand trees and shrubs, representing 325 varieties—more tree varieties than any other urban park in the United States. In its early years, the park had more than ten thousand trees; a reforestation plan may one day enlarge its tree inventory.

In the fall, the gingkos glow yellow. Spring coaxes the dogwoods, magnolias, and ornamental fruit trees into blossom. Summer brings the cool refreshment of leafy shade and the flowering lily pond, and in winter the evergreens sport vivid greens and boughs heavy with snow. Flowering bulbs and floral displays provide colorful beauty from March through October.

Though historic and fanciful, the park begs to be used. The second largest park in the city, Tower Grove has seven miles of trails and roads, almost half of which are closed to cars. Numerous benches, picnic tables, tennis courts, a summer wading pool, and ball fields make this a vital urban area.

This walk covers two miles of trails on the park's eastern side, which is the most ornamental. The western side contains playing fields, a wild bird garden, and some stone stables, which are the park's oldest buildings. You may want to explore this area as well.

In this consummate walking park, pedestrians have the right of way, but watch for traffic when you cross the streets.

The walk

➤Enter the park through the Magnolia Avenue entrance. The stags you see reposing atop the pillars at this gate are made of zinc; each weighs seven hundred pounds. The gate's fifteen-foot limestone columns came from the Old Courthouse when it was remodeled. The park has four intricate stone and iron gates. Their style and interesting embellishments are among the details that mark this park as Victorian.

➤Once inside the gates, take the asphalt path to your right and in front of you.

➤Cross Northwest Drive, which is a one-way road heading to your right, and pick up the path that angles toward the tennis courts. Just past the tennis courts you will see the elaborate playground pavilion, which serves as a backdrop to the large wading pool, swings, and jungle gym.

➤Follow the path as it comes up on the Nos. 1, 2, and 3 grass tennis courts, which are to your left. The wooden climbing gym is on your right.

➤Cross Southwest Drive, which goes one way to your left.

➤Once on the other side of Southwest Drive, turn left on the walking path and go toward the road ahead. On your right you will see the 1888 white stone Arsenal Street Gatehouse; it was one of four built for each of the park's gatekeepers. Designed by George I. Barnett, one of Shaw's favorite architects, it now houses the park offices.

➤Cross Center Cross Drive and turn left. In front of you is the red-and-white-striped Turkish Shelter, a former dovecote that is now popular for family gatherings. Shaw had ten pavilions built in the park that, in his words, would "afford shelter from showers and sunshine." The shelters are scattered throughout the park's east side and were intended to give strollers a place to stop, rest, and view the park's lovely features.

➤Turn right and enter the path that is closed to traffic. This path runs along the other side of the Turkish Shelter. You may want to go inside and look up to its curved roof where birds once roosted.

➤Stay on the path. You will spot the park's many amenities: grills, picnic tables, benches and water fountains.

➤Cross the road at the intersection where you see the blue water fountain and the green road rails and continue on the path. The Old Carriage Shelter, a smaller, ornate pavilion, is on your right.

➤ You will cross a brightly painted foot bridge. This bridge and others cross small waterways that help water the park's trees. At the roundabout, your path will curve slightly to the right. A red, white, and blue shelter is on your right. The bronze statue in the middle is of Alexander von Humboldt, a nineteenth-century explorer and naturalist who was much admired. The statue is one of three created for the park by Ferdinand Miller.

➤Continue on this path that follows Main Drive. After the path curves for the second roundabout, you will see the elaborate Chinese Shelter in red and green coming up on your right. You are approaching the east Grand Boulevard entrance to the park. Two zinc griffins adorn this gate, and another Miller bronze, this one of Christopher Columbus, stands sentry at this entrance.

To your right, in the park's southeast corner, you will see the Stupp Center and Memorial Garden. This is the only senior center set within a park in the state; it is a popular spot for weddings and family reunions.

If it is near the time for lunch, dinner, or just a great snack, you may want to leave Tower Grove Park through this gate and explore the many interesting restaurants and shops along South Grand, which is Walk 8. Turn to page 100 for directions in the area locals call "Grand South Grand." Then resume your park walk on your return.

➤Cross Main Drive in front of Columbus and go to the path on the other side of Main.

➤Turn left and take this path back into the park. You are now walking along the north side of Main Drive. A water fountain and benches will come up on your right, and you will also find a restroom in this area. Note the elaborate shelter accented with blue, white, and gold paint.

➤After you curve around the first roundabout, you will cross another elaborate bridge spanning a tiny waterway. Walk straight ahead.

➤After passing the gold and yellow Humboldt North Shelter, take the path that heads toward the music bandstand. Architect George Barnett also designed the bandstand, which is the site of summer concerts. Busts of famous composers, each set atop a pillar, adorn this area.

➤Cross the large driveway in front of the shelter and walk on the path between the busts of Rossini and Mozart. Go to your left, passing Mozart, Wagner, and Beethoven.

➤Take the path to your left after you pass Beethoven. Off to your left are the ruins and lily ponds. The ruins serve as a dramatic backdrop for the small ponds and were popular additions to Victorian landscaping. Shaw salvaged these stones and columns from the Lindell Hotel when it burned.

➤Circle the statue of Baron Friedrich Wilhelm von Steuben, a Prussian who helped the American forces at Valley Forge. The German government presented this as a gift to the 1904

World's Fair. After passing Steuben, you will come upon a waterway with plants, ducks, and an island. On the right is the Palm House, the oldest greenhouse west of the Mississippi.

➤Go to the end of the sidewalk that comes up after the water garden. The little pavilion off to your left is the Lily Pond Shelter. Just beyond the shelter in the middle of Center Cross Drive is the third Miller bronze, this one of Shakespeare.

➤Turn right and cross Northeast Bikeway.

➤Walk along Center Cross Drive through the gates and out of the park. If you are in a wheelchair or pushing a stroller, you might want to cross Center Cross Drive and walk along the other side of the street to avoid a bump on this side.

walk **8**

Grand South Grand

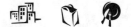

General location: Just southeast of the Missouri Botanical Garden and Tower Grove Park.

Special attractions: Cultural diversity best represented in the shops, groceries, and wonderful ethnic restaurants, especially Asian.

Difficulty rating: Easy, flat, on sidewalks.

Distance: 1 mile.

Estimated time: 30 minutes.

Services: Several restaurants. Restrooms just inside the east entrance of Tower Grove Park at the Stupp Senior Center.

Restrictions: In spite of curb cuts and sidewalks, this walk may be difficult for wheelchair users or those pushing strollers. Traffic is heavy at the intersections.

Grand South Grand

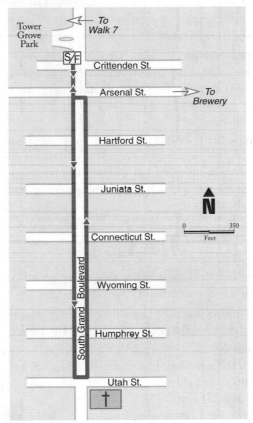

Tower
Grove
Park

To
Walk 7

S/F

Crittenden St.

Arsenal St.

To
Brewery

Hartford St.

Juniata St.

N

0   350
Feet

Connecticut St.

South Grand Boulevard

Wyoming St.

Humphrey St.

Utah St.

For more information: Contact the St. Louis Convention and Visitors Commission or the area restaurants.

Getting started: This walk starts at the east entrance of Tower Grove Park, which exits onto Grand Boulevard. See Walk 7 for more detailed directions on reaching Tower Grove Park.

Grand is a major north-south thoroughfare west of downtown. Interstates 64 and 44 both have exits for Grand. When you exit the interstate, go south on Grand. Park along Grand or a nearby side street.

Public transportation: Bi-State Transit Bus 21 stops at the intersection of Grand and Arsenal, which is not far from the start of this walk. This bus originates at the downtown terminal at Broadway and Locust. Call Bi-State Transit to confirm times.

Overview: South Grand is one of the newest neighborhoods in St. Louis to experience revitalization. Between the 3000 and 3200 blocks of Grand, you will find interesting shops, exotic restaurants, outdoor dining in nice weather, and abundant local color.

The walk

➤As you face the east entrance to Tower Grove Park, turn to your left and walk toward Arsenal.

➤Cross Arsenal carefully. You will have a light, but the traffic turning right onto Arsenal can be heavy and quick.

➤You will walk along this side of Grand for six blocks until you reach the intersection of Grand and Utah Street. Here are the interesting places you most likely will pass along this side of South Grand:

You will find fascinating folk art at Faru Unlimited (#3111). The Mekong Restaurant (#3131) serves Vietnamese food. For traditional bakery goods and scrumptious cakes, stop in Dickmann's Boulevard Bakery (#3139). You will find delicious Thai food at the King & I (#3157). At Holyland Meat and Bakery (#3173), look closely at the address—it is written in Arabic.

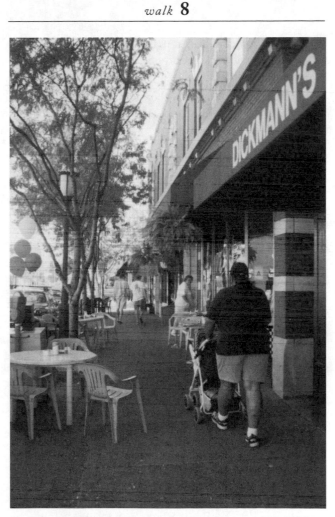

Patio dining, interesting shops, and good restaurants are part of the scene on South Grand Boulevard.

➤When you come to Utah, turn to your left and cross Grand with the light. St. Pius V Catholic Church is at the corner to your right.

➤Now walk north along the other side of Grand. Keep your eyes peeled for interesting shops and eateries. Here are some of the places you may see on this side of South Grand:

The Da Nang restaurant serves Vietnamese food. The Siete Mares (#3204) specializes in Nicaraguan cuisine. Its nacatamal is similar to a Mexican tamale, but it is wrapped in a steamed banana leaf filled with pork, green peppers, rice, tomatoes, raisins, and olives. The Jay Asia Food Co. (#3172) is a full-service Asian grocery that is fun to explore.

➤When you reach Arsenal, turn to your left and cross Grand with the light.

➤Then cross Arsenal with the light, watching for traffic entering the turn lane in front of you.

➤Walk alongside Tower Grove Park until you reach the park's east gate.

If you interrupted your Tower Grove Park walk to explore South Grand, return to the Christopher Columbus statue and the rest of your walk. If you have not yet started the Tower Grove Park walk, turn to page 90. You will find both a map and directions that will help you start this walk from the east gate.

walk 9

Soulard

General location: Just south of downtown.

Special attractions: Quaint neighborhood with nineteenth-century architecture; oldest, continuously operating farmer's market; Anheuser-Busch Brewery, great restaurants and live music.

Difficulty rating: Easy, flat, on sidewalks.

Distance: 2.5 miles—or 4 miles if you add on tours of Soulard Market and the Anheuser-Busch Brewery.

Estimated time: 1 to 3 hours.

Services: Several restaurants, Soulard Market, visitor services at brewery tour center.

Restrictions: Soulard Market is open Wednesday through Saturday. Neither the market nor Busch Brewery are wheelchair-accessible. Not all establishments along this walk have

Soulard

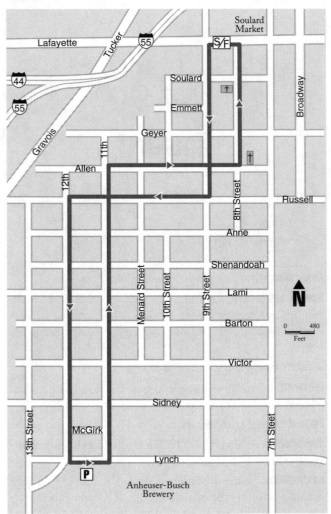

wheelchair-accessible restrooms. Most of the sidewalks have curb cuts, but ongoing restoration in this area may mean some sidewalks could, at times, be roped off or broken.

For more information: Contact the St. Louis Convention and Visitors Commission, Soulard Market, or the Anheuser-Busch Brewery.

Getting started: This walk begins on the bricked plaza in front of the south entrance of Soulard Market. The market is at the corner of 7th Street and Lafayette Avenue. From downtown, take Broadway south. At Park Avenue, 7th merges into Broadway just off to your right. Follow 7th for another block and watch for the market, which will come up on your right. Turn right on Lafayette and look for a parking spot along the side streets. Check parking signs carefully; illegally parked cars may be towed.

Public transportation: Bi-State Transit Bus 99 stops at the corner of Lafayette and 7th Street. Buses 3, 40 and 73 go to the Anheuser-Busch Brewery. The brewery is at the southernmost point of this walk and could serve as a start point for those who want to begin their walk at the brewery. Contact Bi-State Transit to confirm routes and times.

Overview: Stalls piled high with fresh fruits and vegetables, buckets of colorful and fragrant flowers, bags of pungent spices and aromatic coffees, whiffs of smoked sausages and fresh donuts, the cackle of hens, and the shouts of vendors vying for customers—Soulard Market is an eye-popping, nose-tingling, and wallet-friendly adventure. One of the oldest city markets in the country, it has been in continuous operation on this spot since 1779.

The market is named for Antoine P. Soulard, a former French naval lieutenant and King's Surveyor for upper Louisiana. His widow, Madame Julie Soulard, gave this land to the city on the condition that it always be used as a market place. It was here that a struggling young farmer named Ulysses S. Grant came to sell the cord wood that helped him support his family.

The early market buildings were destroyed in an 1896 tornado that devastated this area. When it was rebuilt, the south entrance was modeled after the Foundling Hospital of Florence, Italy. Built in 1419, the hospital is considered the first building created in true Renaissance style.

The market is at the heart of a neighborhood filled with church steeples, brick sidewalks, and interesting architectural details like black wrought-iron accents and mansard roofs. Soulard Neighborhood is on the National Register of Historic Places because of the quantity and quality of its older buildings—many of them in the Federal and French Second Empire styles of the 1800s.

Like so many neighborhoods near downtown, Soulard has seen extensive renovation and restoration. This renewal has brought with it some great restaurants and a live music scene that makes this area one of the city's hottest night spots.

The area really comes alive on July 14—Bastille Day— and again for Mardi Gras during the two weeks preceding Lent. Revelers come to Soulard to enjoy wine tastings, balls, art shows, bike races, and a parade that attracts about 100,000 masked party-goers.

The walk

➤This walk starts on the sidewalk in front of Soulard Market's south entrance. If the market is open, plan to start or end your walk with a trip through the interior. The market has a central corridor that includes a bakery, butcher,

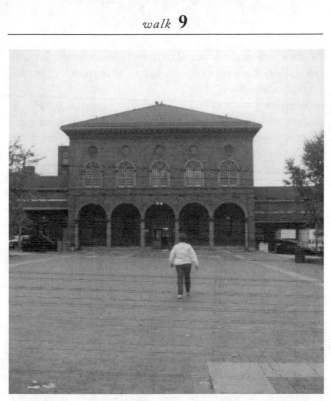

The newest entrance to Soulard Market was built in 1928 in the Italian Renaissance style.

spice shop, and restrooms. Four shopping hallways filled with vendor stalls jut out from either side of the central hall-way. A complete circuit covers about half a mile. The market is liveliest on Saturday.

➤At the sidewalk by Lafayette Avenue, with your back to the market, turn right and walk along Lafayette to 9th Street.

➤Turn left at 9th and cross Lafayette. You will walk along 9th for five blocks. At 9th and Soulard, your first intersection, stands a lone house. Before urban blight struck Soulard, the area was densely populated and almost every lot was used. Today the empty spaces are all that were left by the wrecking ball.

With its shuttered houses, wrought-iron trims, tiny back gardens and patios, and narrow buildings with even narrower passageways, this neighborhood looks and feels a bit like New Orleans, which is not surprising since this city had strong, early ties to Louisiana and southern French culture.

Patty Long's Ninth Street Abbey at #1808 is an interesting example of creative reuse, for this former church is now a restaurant and bar. It has a wheelchair-accessible entrance, parking, and restrooms.

When you reach Geyer Avenue, you are close to two popular live music spots. At the corner of 9th and Geyer, you will find the 1860s Saloon and Hard Shell Cafe, which showcases blues and dancing nightly. Mike & Min's at 925 Geyer is considered the city's blues mecca.

➤At Russell Boulevard, turn right and walk to 12th St. Russell is a little wider and busier, with more stores, a few taverns, and a pizzeria. Watch for #1009 on your side of the street, and look toward its upper windows for a terra-cotta milkmaid and her two cows.

➤At 12th turn left and cross Russell with the light. Look for John D. McGurk's Irish Pub at 1200 Russell. This lively pub features Ireland's best musicians and beer.

As you walk toward Lynch Street, you will pass through a slightly more elegant neighborhood. Built on higher ground, the homes along 12th were bought by those who could afford a finer view of the city. Be sure to look up to the roofs where you will find an array of turrets, chimneys, dormers nestled into sloping mansard roofs, and ornamental trimmings.

At Sidney Street and 12th, be sure to notice the corner house built in the octagon style. All along the way, look for set-in doorways, some with distinctive painting, others with carved doors, still others with a concrete lion standing guard. As you approach Lynch, an art deco police station will come up across the street on your right.

➤Cross Lynch and turn left. You will see the visitor entrance to the Anheuser-Busch Brewery and may catch the strong aroma of hops. This historic brewery is the only one remaining in a neighborhood that once had several. If you want a tour, go into the parking lot and follow the signs toward the Tour Center. Each tour takes about ninety minutes and ends with complimentary samples of Busch beers.

➤Go to the intersection of 11th Street and Lynch. The Lynch Street Bistro is on the corner. This restaurant not only has good food in a beautifully renovated space, but also several original paintings by William S. Burroughs, the Beat novelist.

➤At 11th turn left. You will walk several blocks down this residential street on your way to Allen Avenue. As you pass through this neighborhood, note the homes undergoing renovation, as well as those that obviously have been reclaimed. Once again keep on the lookout for interesting architectural details.

➤Cross Russell carefully, for you will not have a light and the oncoming traffic does not have a stop sign.

➤After crossing Allen, which is one block past Russell, turn right and continue to 8th Street.

➤Cross 8th and turn left. You are now in front of Saints Peter and Paul Catholic Church.

Founded in 1849, Saints Peter and Paul once had four thousand parishioners and was among the most significant

German Catholic parishes in the country. By the 1960s, urban flight had reduced the parish rolls to less than four hundred.

If it is open, look inside the church for its mix of the traditional and the unconventional. The traditional stained glass windows, which were made in Innsbrook, Austria, and

of interest

The Busch tour

Offered Monday through Saturday, the ninety-minute, free Anheuser-Busch Brewery tour is fascinating and well worth your time. A brief film at the start offers details on the brewing process, the Anheuser and Busch families, and the beer empire they created. The recently renovated Brew House, the paddock of the famous Clydesdales, and the interesting and often elegant architectural details will capture your interest and imagination.

Some things to consider before you commit to the tour: This is a popular tourist attraction, so depending on the time of year, you might be assigned to a tour group that leaves an hour or more from when you enter the visitor center.

Brewing requires both hot and chilly temperatures, so be prepared for sharp temperature fluctuations. Also, while on the tour, you will walk about a mile on the grounds and in some buildings will go up and down several stairs. But when you have covered the sights, a tram stands ready to take you back to the hospitality room.

People pushing strollers or walking with young children should bypass the brewery tour. Instead, visit Grants Farm—another free Busch attraction south of the city—which will delight anyone who loves wild animals, handsome horses, and a country setting.

If you take the brewery tour, return to the parking lot entrance on Lynch Street to resume this walk.

the back of the altar are original to the church, which was built in the late 1800s. The oil-painted Stations of the Cross come from Germany and are among only three such sets in the world and the only set in the United States.

The church's unconventional appearance rests in its pew arrangement. Instead of neatly aligned from front to back, the pews are arranged near the altar in a theater-in-the-round style. Today Saints Peter and Paul ministers to hundreds of the city's homeless. Its unique interior reflects the changes this parish has witnessed, for both this church and the Soulard neighborhood have experienced decline and dramatic rebirth.

After you pass the church and cross into the next block, take a moment to hunt for a "mousetrap!" In this neighborhood, a mousetrap is a tunnel-like corridor that goes through a house and gives access to the house's other floors and areas. You will find a good example at #1808.

At the corner of Soulard and 8th, you will find Trinity Lutheran Church. This historic building was originally built in 1864 and partially rebuilt after the 1896 tornado. The oldest Lutheran Church west of the Mississippi, it is the home church for the Lutheran Church, Missouri Synod, and is open for public tours and workshops.

➤Continue down 8th until your walk ends where you started, at the front of Soulard Market.

From Soulard you are only a short distance from the walk at Lafayette Square on page 118 or a walk among the antique shops of Cherokee Street on page 112. To reach the Lafayette walk, take Lafayette Avenue west to Lafayette Park. If you want to walk along Cherokee, take Lafayette to Jefferson Avenue and turn left. See these walks for more detailed directions.

walk 10
Cherokee Street

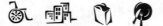

General location: Just south of Anheuser-Busch Brewery.

Special attractions: Historic district, antique stores, DeMenil and Lemp mansions, quaint neighborhood.

Difficulty rating: Easy, flat, and entirely on sidewalks.

Distance: 1 mile.

Estimated time: 30 minutes.

Services: Restaurants and shops.

Restrictions: Most stores and restaurants are open between Wednesday and Saturday. Many places, including the Chatillon-DeMenil Mansion, are closed Mondays. Restrooms are available only to customers, and few, if any, are wheelchair accessible.

For more information: Contact the St. Louis Convention and Visitors Commission.

Cherokee Street

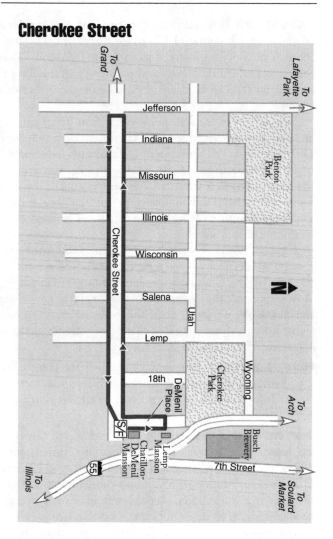

Getting started: This walk starts at the Chatillon-DeMenil Mansion at the corner of Cherokee Street and DeMenil Place. You will find metered parking on DeMenil Place; the meters take only nickels and quarters, and the limit is two hours. You can also park along Cherokee or other side streets.

You can get to the start point either from Jefferson Avenue on the western edge of the Cherokee-Lemp Historic District or from 7th Street on its eastern edge. Jefferson is a major north/south street and the downtown's western border. Take Jefferson south. After you pass Arsenal Street, look for the street-lamp sign for Cherokee Antique Row and the DeMenil Mansion. Turn left on Cherokee and go eight blocks to the mansion.

If you come via 7th Street, go south past the Anheuser-Busch Brewery. Just when it seems 7th will end, you will see the sign for the Chatillon-DeMenil Mansion. Turn right. As you approach the mansion, take the street that goes along the mansion's side. Do not take the road that curves to your right in front of the mansion; this is an entrance ramp to Interstate 55.

Public transportation: You can pick up Bi-State Transit Bus 20 downtown and take it to Cherokee Street. Contact Bi-State's Information Center for times, the exact route, and fares.

Overview: Once a working-class neighborhood of tiny two-story, red-brick houses, front-porch stoops, varied storefronts, and tree-lined streets, the Cherokee-Lemp Historic District is now home to St. Louis's most famous antique district. Here you will find everything from ordinary household utensils, to vintage radios and Victrolas, antique chandeliers and lighting, Victorian hardware, war mementos, old furniture, toys, stained glass, antique books, and tons of

114

bric-a-brac and collectibles. You will also find a few restaurants on Cherokee that serve sandwiches and beverages. The mansions' restaurants offer more elegant fare.

Take time to peek in the many shop windows and to appreciate these solid, modest houses. Many of the shops are located in homes that once belonged to the German immigrants who worked in the area's breweries. This trendy area is seeing a resurgence, and many of the newly refurbished buildings reflect this area's urban rebirth.

The walk

Begin your walk in front of Chatillon-DeMenil Mansion.

➤Walk in front of the mansion and away from Cherokee Street.

➤Stop in front of the Lemp Mansion, which is just next door. After you have studied this grand old home, look behind the house and to your left for the church spires of St. Agatha's Catholic Church, which is a historic landmark.

➤Cross DeMenil Place and walk along the four-flat apartments back to Cherokee Street.

➤Turn right on Cherokee. You now will walk eight blocks along this side of Cherokee. Most often the cars traveling the side streets have stop signs, but be watchful of traffic at the corners.

Shortly after you start this walk, look for the Lemp brewery buildings, which will come up on your left. If you are hungry or thirsty, look for the Cherokee Coffee Co., which will come up on your right at 2013 Cherokee.

➤At Jefferson Avenue, turn left and cross Cherokee, then turn left again and walk along the other side of Cherokee. If you enjoy imagining the way things were many years ago,

of interest

Some mansion history

The Chatillon-DeMenil Mansion is one of the city's finest specimens of Greek Revival architecture. You can tour the mansion, where you will find historic portraits and furnishings, a gift shop, and a restaurant in the carriage house.

The section of the house that faces DeMenil Place was built in 1848 for Henri Chatillon, who had worked as a frontier guide. His home resembled a farmhouse instead of the mansion it would later become under Dr. Nicholas DeMenil. When DeMenil expanded the house, he incorporated the Greek Revival characteristics that can be seen from Interstate 55. Members of the DeMenil family lived here until 1929.

In the early 1960s, when Interstate 55 cut a wide swath through the neighborhood, the house was spared, but only by a matter of feet. An interstate on-ramp comes so close to the mansion's stately columns that the ramp almost appears to be the mansion's curving driveway.

The Lemp Mansion, now a restaurant and bed and breakfast, is said to be haunted by members of the Lemp family. This ill-fated brewing family had its start with William J. Lemp, who imported fine European craftsmen to embellish this home. A German immigrant, Lemp introduced lager beer to an appreciative public. It was estimated that from March to September in 1854, St. Louisans quaffed 18 million glasses of lager, stopping only when they drank the supply dry.

Prohibition forced the brewery to liquidate, and the family suffered several personal tragedies—no one survived to carry on the name. All that remains of this once popular brewery are its buildings, which you will see at the start of this walk, and the family's mausoleum in Bellefontaine Cemetery.

imagine Jefferson Avenue in the late 1700s. The street marks the western edge of the common fields that the city founders established for the common foraging, agriculture, and grazing that sustained the young community. Cows once roamed where cars and pedestrians now vie for space.

➤When you reach DeMenil and Cherokee, cross Cherokee and return to your car.

Would you like to explore other historic neighborhoods in this area? You are within a short drive of the Soulard Market walk, which starts on page 103, or the walk around Lafayette Park, which starts on page 118. If you want to tour the Anheuser-Busch Brewery, this area's neighbor to the north, turn to Appendix B on page 219 for information about these tours or to page 110 for information about the brewery and its history.

walk 11
Lafayette Square

General location: A little west and south of downtown and a few miles north of Anheuser-Busch Brewery.

Special attractions: Restored neighborhood, nineteenth-century Victorian homes, city's oldest public park, "private places."

Difficulty rating: Easy, flat, all on sidewalks.

Distance: 0.75 mile—or 1.25 miles if you explore the park.

Estimated time: 30 minutes.

Services: No restaurants or shops on streets bordering the park. Restaurants in the vicinity of Park Avenue and 18th Street.

Restrictions: Dogs must be leashed and their droppings picked up.

For more information: Contact Lafayette House Bed and Breakfast or the St. Louis Convention and Visitors Commission.

Lafayette Square

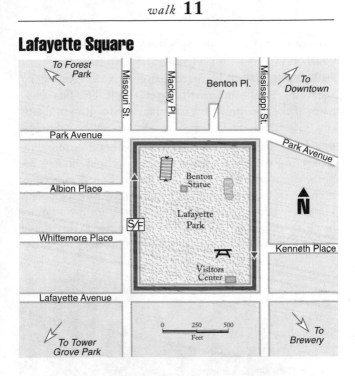

To Forest Park

Missouri St.

Mackay Pl.

Benton Pl.

Mississippi St.

To Downtown

Park Avenue

Park Avenue

Albion Place

Benton Statue

Whittemore Place

S/F

Lafayette Park

Kenneth Place

Visitors Center

Lafayette Avenue

N

0 250 500
Feet

To Tower Grove Park

To Brewery

Getting started: You can start anywhere on one of the sidewalks that border Lafayette Park. This walk goes completely around the park, with side options to explore the park and to visit Benton Place, the city's oldest surviving "private place." The walking directions start on Missouri Street between Lafayette and Park avenues. If you start from another location, check the map to orient yourself with the walk's text.

If coming toward the city by interstate, take I-44—the closest to Lafayette Park—east toward downtown. Take Exit 289 at Jefferson Avenue. Take Jefferson north one block to Lafayette and turn to your right. Lafayette Park and

Missouri Street will come up quickly on your left. Turn left on Missouri and park your car.

Public transportation: Bi-State Transit Bus 99 travels along Lafayette Avenue and past Lafayette Park. This bus originates at the downtown bus terminal at Broadway and Locust. Contact Bi-State Transit to confirm routes and times.

Overview: Lafayette Square, the neighborhood surrounding Lafayette Park, has experienced glory, decline, and now rebirth. Within the western boundary of St. Louis's early common lands, the area attracted the city's wealthiest citizens. Here they built elegant two- and three-story town homes in what was then the suburbs. The elite partied in their grand houses and strolled Lafayette Park undisturbed by outsiders.

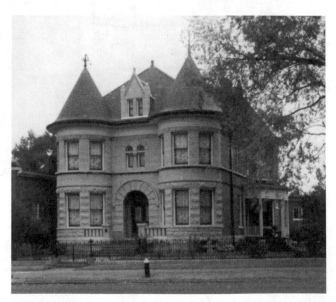

This grand home at 2031 Park survived a tornado in 1896.

As the city grew beyond Lafayette Square, the neighborhood's prominent residents withdrew to even more private places in the West End. The area lost its exclusive appeal, and the devastating tornado of 1896 set in motion the neighborhood's dramatic decline. By the 1940s, Lafayette Square had joined the list of blighted neighborhoods. Rumors in the 1950s of impending highway construction made residents hesitant to repair homes that might be bulldozed.

In the late 1960s and early 1970s, new people—lured by incredibly cheap prices for homes with incredible potential— began to fill the vacant houses in Lafayette Square. In 1972, the area became the city's first historical district, and today it has recaptured its sense of elegance and charm. Its new residents, like its original ones, are professional people with resources who find in this urban setting a sense of peace and escape from the city's bustle.

The walk

On Missouri Street, between Park and Lafayette avenues, take a moment to study the grand homes on Lafayette Park's western border. The 1896 tornado struck hardest the area at the corner of Lafayette and Missouri, leveling the homes and then demolishing the park. The large Romanesque mansions you see on this block replaced the homes that were destroyed.

➤With the park on your right, walk toward Park Avenue.

➤Turn right on Park. Look across the street at the row of ornate houses painted in the colorful Victorian style. Splashes of turquoise, rust, yellow, and blue reflect the Victorian taste for intricate house painting.

Look across the street for 2115 Park with its ornately carved door and marble columns. At 2031 Park you will

Explore Lafayette Park

Lafayette Park has several entrances and many winding paths, so any time during your walk, take a moment to stroll inside this lovely, thirty-acre park. You will not have any trouble finding your way out of the park or back to your car.

This park not only is St. Louis's oldest park, it is also the only common land remaining from the land Pierre Laclède set aside for common use. What you cannot see well or at all from the sidewalk are the park's gardens; tiny Lafayette Lake with swans, ducks, and geese who look like they expect to be fed; picnic tables and benches; the bandstand, where the summer concert series is held; a par course fitness circuit; and two statues—one of George Washington and the other of Thomas Hart Benton, one of Missouri's first two U.S. senators.

Benton came to St. Louis in 1815 and soon became editor of the *St. Louis Enquirer*. For almost thirty years, he promoted St. Louis as the city that could play a major role in world trade. He fought for a railroad line that would connect St. Louis with San Francisco and the Pacific. This ocean port would be the Midwest's access to the riches of the Far East and the "China Trade." When you find Benton's statue toward the middle of the park, look for the inscription on the pedestal: ". . .there is the East! there is India!" It speaks to Benton's trading dream for St. Louis.

Today the Benton bronze is surrounded by trees and gardens. But after the 1896 tornado, the statue stood amidst devastation, a solitary survivor in the path of destruction. The tornado, which killed more than one hundred people and injured more than one thousand, did its worst damage between this park and the Mississippi River.

Connecting to other walks

If you are driving, Lafayette Street can be a major route for reaching other walks. You can take Lafayette east to the Soulard Market walk, which starts at Lafayette and 7th Street. You can also return to downtown by turning left on 7th, which will become Broadway before you reach downtown.

You can get to the Cherokee Street walk and the antique stores by taking Lafayette west to Jefferson. Turn left at Jefferson and follow it for a little over a mile to Cherokee, where you will turn left.

To get to the three walks in the Tower Grove Park area, including the Missouri Botanical Garden walk, take Lafayette west to Grand Avenue. Turn left on Grand, go one block, and turn right on Shaw, which leads to the gardens.

If you are traveling by bus and would like to visit other walks, catch Bus 99 on Lafayette. This bus stops at 7th and Lafayette at the Soulard Market. It also connects to the downtown walks; the walks at the Missouri Botanical Garden, Tower Grove Park and Grand South Grand; and the neighborhood Hill walk. Call Bi-State Transit to confirm the exact routes and times.

find a grand home designed by Theodore Link, the architect who designed Union Station. This home of turrets with finials, detailed stone work and arched entryway was completed the day the tornado struck. It survived virtually intact.

Still across the street and a little farther down, you will see the entrance to Benton Place, at the corner of Benton Place and Park. St. Louis is known for its "private places," the lovely, exceedingly private residential streets that were

of interest

Private places

The gated streets, or "private places," you find in St. Louis are unique to this city. Started in the late 1800s by city surveyor Julius Pitzman, they were designed to protect the city's wealthy from the inconvenience of city life—noise, traffic, pollution, and unnecessary mixing with people they would not invite to dinner.

Private places were governed by common deed restrictions. The residents maintained the streets, and entrance gates at either end and plantings down the streets' centers slowed or stopped traffic. Even today, private places have only one entrance for cars. Found throughout the central city, these places are most concentrated in the Central West End, primarily between Union Boulevard and either side of Kingshighway.

Pitzman designed forty-seven private places, and over time they popped up farther and farther west of the city. Their birth and decline chart the migration of the city's well-to-do from city life to suburban living. Isaac Lionberger, a prominent nineteenth-century businessman noted that "those who have the means move continually, leaving behind what they cannot endure." Today, many of the city's wealthiest residents have moved once again, this time to private estates in Ladue, just west of the city limits.

Lovely and protected, even in their declining years, the private places of St. Louis never completely succumbed to urban blight. Instead, they patiently waited to be reclaimed even as their market values plummeted. Their rebirth came with the return of people who loved the city, who wanted to live within its urban core, and who could afford faded beauty. These returnees and the homes they lovingly restored have given St. Louis something most cities cannot create—elegant, vital neighborhoods in the heart of the city.

closed to through traffic. Benton Place is the oldest of these private places.

If you wish to explore this area, carefully cross Park now, or go to the corner of Park and Mississippi Street and double back. Inside Benton Place you will find several lovely homes arranged around a shaded center oval and an overall feel of renewal and restoration. Then return to this spot.

➤Continue down Park to Mississippi Street.

➤Turn right onto Mississippi. Once again the park is to your right and a row of older homes is across the street. Narrow, but deep, these homes are sometimes separated by the narrowest of walkways. These houses are even more colorful than their Park Street neighbors. Who can miss the lime-green house with yellow-green trim or the yellow house with salmon and orange trimmings?

If you are curious about these homes—what they have inside or what they sell for—look for 1552 Mississippi, the blue house with pink trim. In 1997, this house was listed for sale at $156,000. Although it may not look especially grand from the outside, this Greek Revival style home has eleven rooms. Its features include high ceilings, twin parlors, parquet flooring, a dramatic staircase, a paneled library/billiard room, functional gas fireplaces in almost every room, and a grand entrance hall with pocket doors. Remodeled for today's tastes, it also includes a Jacuzzi room and master bedroom, second-floor laundry room, updated kitchen, walk-out decks and a three-car garage!

➤Turn right at the intersection of Mississippi and Lafayette. As you walk along this side of the park, look across the street for 2156 Lafayette, a large Queen Anne. Captain James Eads, the designer and builder of St. Louis's Eads Bridge, had this home built for his daughter as a wedding present.

Today the home is a bed-and-breakfast inn known as Lafayette House.

On your side of Lafayette you will pass the neighborhood's original and quaint police station. Built in 1867, it is now a visitors center.

➤At the intersection of Lafayette and Missouri, turn right and return to your car.

walk **12**

University City

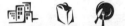

General location: Northwest of Forest Park on the Washington University Hilltop Campus and in nearby University City at the city's western limits.

Special attractions: Major university campus, World's Fair sites, "private places," the Loop, and the Walk of Fame.

Difficulty rating: Easy, on sidewalks, with some stairs.

Distance: 3.5 miles.

Estimated time: 2 hours.

Services: Restrooms on campus and along route, information center and theater in the Student Union Building.

Restrictions: On campus, dogs must be on leashes no longer than six feet. Some campus buildings are closed weekends.

For more information: Contact the St. Louis Convention and Visitors Commission or Washington University.

University City

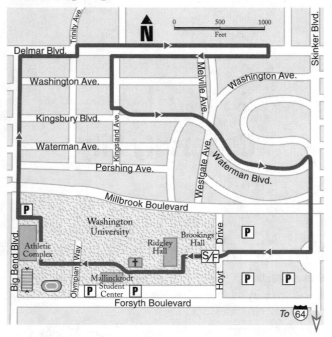

Getting started: Interstates 64 and 170 come within a few miles of Washington University. From I-64, take the McCausland exit and turn north. McCausland turns into Skinker Boulevard. The university will be a mile down and on the left. Turn left on Brookings Drive. From I-170, go south to the Forest Park Parkway exit. Go about two miles east on the parkway to Skinker. Turn right and then quickly turn right again at Brookings Drive. Visitor parking is on either side of Brookings Drive. Meters take quarters only. Four quarters buy the maximum, which is two hours, but ticketing reportedly is lax in this lot.

128

Public transportation: This campus is well-served by public transportation. Bi-State Transit Bus 97 stops along Big Bend Boulevard, where you can intersect with the walk on page 133. Bus 93 travels on Skinker in front of Brookings Hall, the walk's start. The yellow-and-black Shuttle Bee picks up commuters at the Forest Park MetroLink station and passes by Washington University along Millbrook Boulevard. Call Bi-State Transit to confirm routes and schedules. The university also runs a Medical School shuttle bus that stops at the Central West End and the Forest Park MetroLink stations. Stand by the white, red, and green signs outside the stations, flag the bus down, and tell the driver you want to get off at Brookings Hall. The shuttle runs year round.

Overview: You will walk not only on the Washington University campus, but also along Delmar Boulevard and through The Loop, University City's popular student and tourist area. The Loop, which runs for four blocks on either side of Delmar, takes its name from an old streetcar turnaround. It takes its feel, however, from the funky restaurants and music venues, and from the street cafes, bookstores, record shops, and art galleries so often associated with urban college life.

Like the main street of any college town, Delmar bustles with shoppers and diners. The hungry can dig into classic American hamburgers and fries and microbrewed root beer, but international cuisine also simmers in these restaurant kitchens. Here you will find fare from Lebanon, Thailand, Greece, Japan, and Ethiopia. On the weekends, many of the bars and restaurants also hop to the beat of live music.

Remember to look down as you walk along Delmar, for you will find the St. Louis Walk of Fame beneath your feet. Brass stars and plaques embedded in the sidewalk honor actors, athletes, or humanitarians who all have one thing in common—they came from St. Louis.

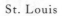

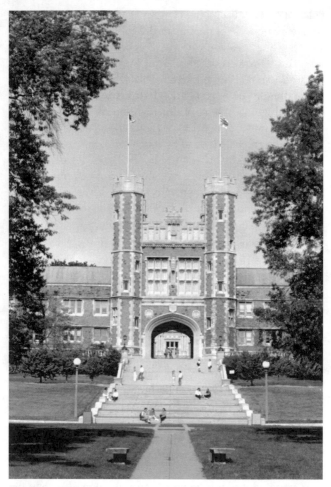

Brookings Hall welcomes visitors to Washington University. Photo courtesy of Washington University.

The walk

➤This walk starts at the grand staircase heading up to Brookings Hall, the administration building for Washington University, known as Wash U. This impressive Collegiate Gothic structure was named for Robert S. Brookings, a wholesale merchant who helped the university leave its cramped downtown space and move to its new campus on the city's western limit. Brookings's walkway emblem notes that "Those who come nearest to truth come nearest to God."

➤Walk through the archway at Brookings Hall and into Brookings Quadrangle.

➤Walk down the center walkway through the quadrangle. The building directly in front of you is Ridgley Hall.

➤When you reach Ridgley, turn left and follow the sidewalk to the end of the building.

➤Turn right through the archways. A sign points toward Eads Hall, which houses the Undergraduate Admissions Office. You have now entered a smaller quadrangle.

➤Follow the tree-lined path that stretches in front of you. Eads Hall is to your right. The modern building also on your right and just beyond Eads is the Olin Library, built in the 1960s. On your left is Charles Rebstock Hall. The next building on your right after the library is Graham Chapel. The sidewalk angling off to your left just before you reach the chapel leads to Mallinckrodt Student Center, the Edison Theatre and Campus Bookstore. You will find restrooms and food in the student center, as well as a good bookstore and information about upcoming theater offerings.

➤Walk to the main entrance of Graham Chapel and go inside. Modeled after King's College Chapel in Cambridge, England, the chapel is a venue for concerts and lectures as

St. Louis

of interest

Washington University

Washington University began life in 1853 as Eliot Seminary and was named for one of its founders, William Greenleaf Eliot, a Unitarian minister. In 1857, the school changed its name to Washington University. Even then it was highly regarded for its non-denominational, even liberal, approach to higher education.

First located downtown, Wash U moved to its present site at the turn of the century. In 1904, the university crossed paths with the World's Fair, its short-term neighbor to the east. The university's leaders seized the chance to lease ten of the university's new and still unoccupied buildings to the fair and to pour the rents back into more construction. So, before Brookings Hall was the school's administrative building, it was the fair's.

The World's Fair closed on December 1, 1904, and about one month later the university opened for business on its new campus. But city historians note that students and faculty reclaimed what looked like a war zone and what sounded like a construction site. About twenty of the fair's temporary buildings on and near campus were still being torn down; rubble was piled everywhere. The Pike, the fair's popular amusement strip, loomed large but silent across from Brookings Hall.

Today, Forest Park, the old fair site, provides a lush border to the eastern edge of Wash U's 169-acre Hilltop Campus, the site of this walk. Its 59-acre Medical Campus is just east of Forest Park in the Central West End. About 11,600 students attend the university. That 84 percent of them come from outside Missouri suggests the school has a strong national reputation.

well as a worship space. Note the stained glass, the arches, the elaborate organ piping, and the chapel's old-world feel.

➤Follow the tree-lined path that leads away from the chapel and through the largest of the campus's grassy plazas.

➤Cross Olympian Way. Directly to your left is Francis Field, the site of the 1904 Olympics. Most of the track and field events were held at this field, and nearly two-thirds of the grandstand on the track's south side is original.

These Olympics were the first held in America and only the third held in modern times. They also were the last Olympics in which athletes came to the games as individuals and not as representatives of their countries.

In 1914 the field was named for David R. Francis, a former Missouri governor and president of the Louisiana Purchase Exposition, the fair's formal name. Francis was instrumental in organizing the 1904 World's Fair and in getting the Olympics to St. Louis.

➤Follow the path as it parallels Francis Field. You are walking toward the Athletic Complex, which was built in 1985.

➤Turn right and take the path that goes in front of the two bears. The Athletic Complex is open Monday through Friday, so you can use the restrooms or drinking fountains on these days.

➤Continue down the path. The Tao Tennis Center will be on your right.

➤Follow the path between the Athletic Complex and the two fraternity houses and toward the parking lot. Just past the lion statues, the sidewalk curves to your left and heads into a parking lot.

➤Turn left into the lot and follow the path to the stairs.

➤Go down the stairs and turn right—the only way you can go.

➤At the end, turn left. You are out of the university complex and standing along Big Bend Boulevard.

Note: If you have taken Bus 97, you will connect with the walk's route here.

➤Turn right and walk along Big Bend. On your left you will find attractive housing.

➤Cross Millbrook Boulevard. On your right you will find gated neighborhoods with their entrances off Delmar.

➤Cross Kingsbury Boulevard. Note the interesting tile and slate roofs of the elegant homes in the private place to your right. The last gated entrance is for University Heights #2.

➤At Delmar, turn right. You are approaching an interesting complex of buildings known as Holy Corners because of the religious and fraternal organizations once located here. The two large pillars decorated with lions and the flower-filled median adds to the area's imposing feel.

A former Masonic Temple is directly across the street on the northwest corner. On the southeast corner, you will find the St. Louis Conservatory and School for the Arts housed in a former synagogue.

The unusual building across the street on the northeast corner was the headquarters for The Woman's Magazine, which was started by Edward Lewis, who founded not only a magazine, but also University City. In 1930, the building became University City's City Hall.

➤Cross Trinity.

➤At the stoplight, which serves Harvard Avenue, cross to the other side of Delmar and go to your right. You will get a closer look at City Hall, which houses murals and a lovely staircase. You will also pass the University City Library.

➤Cross Kingsland Avenue with the light, keeping an eye out for traffic turning onto Kingsland. You are now entering the shopping and dining area known as The Loop. You will find the first Walk of Fame star, which remembers Dred and Harriet Scott, in front of the St. Louis Bread Company. This was the first store for this popular restaurant chain that serves fresh bread, bagels, pastries, and hearty soups. This is also the first of many restaurants you will encounter on Delmar. In the summer, a farmer's market will be just off to your left.

➤Continue along Delmar, taking time to read the star histories and peek in the shop windows.

➤Cross Westgate Avenue. Keep an eye out for the signs marking the city limit.

➤At the point where Delmar intersects the city limit, cross Delmar. You will not have a light, so cross carefully.

➤Once across, turn right and continue down the south side of Delmar. The first star you encounter on this side is for author Kate Chopin. Musician Miles Davis has a star in front of Streetside Records.

In this first block you will also pass the Tivoli Theatre, a restored movie house specializing in art films. Betty Grable's star is in front of the ticket booth.

➤Cross Westgate. At the corner of Westgate and Delmar you will find Blueberry Hill, a restaurant that has become as famous for its atmosphere and jukebox as it has for its hearty sandwich fare and live music. *Cash Box* magazine calls the restaurant's Wurlitzer "the Best Juke Box in America." No doubt your favorites are among its two thousand tunes. Appropriately enough, rock-n-roll great Chuck Berry's star rests at the entrance.

Blueberry Hill is open daily, so step inside, grab a booth or play some darts, soak up the atmosphere, and check out the many collectibles—paraphernalia from Howdy Doody, Pee Wee Herman, the Beatles, Batman, album covers, lunch boxes, baseball cards, comic books, and more. Since it opened in 1972, Blueberry Hill clearly has become a home for Baby Boomer miscellany. In February, the restaurant hosts the annual Elvis Birthday Celebration, complete with guitar-shaped birthday cakes, an Elvis impersonator contest, and live music.

➤Continue down Delmar to Kingsland.

➤Cross Kingsland. At the corner, in Epstein Plaza, you will find the engaging sculpture *Rain Main*, by Gregory Cullen.

➤Turn left on the sidewalk that goes past the post office, which will be on your right. You are entering one of the area's private places, so enjoy the homes and gardens.

➤Cross Washington Avenue.

➤At Kingsbury Boulevard, the next block, turn left and cross Kingsland. In the summer, this shady boulevard will protect you from the sun.

➤Continue down Kingsbury and walk through the wrought-iron gate that blocks car traffic from the private place.

➤When you come to the Y intersection of Washington and Waterman Avenues, take Waterman, the right leg of the Y. Along this avenue, you will find striking older homes, and spacious and well-tended gardens. In the spring, the azalea and rhododendron will be in bloom.

➤Follow Waterman to the exit gate at Skinker Boulevard.

➤After you walk through the stone pillars, turn right and walk along Skinker. Grace Methodist Church is across Skinker.

➤Cross Millbrook Boulevard, which is called Forest Park Parkway on the east side on Skinker.

➤Continue to Brookings Drive, turn right, and return to your car. If you started this walk near the bus stop on Big Bend, turn to the start of this walk and proceed up the staircase to Brookings Hall.

walk 13

Central West End

General location: West of downtown and adjacent to Forest Park.

Special attractions: The Cathedral Basilica of Saint Louis and the world's largest collection of mosaics; distinctive architecture and turn-of-the-century neighborhoods; eclectic shops, galleries, antique stores, and eateries; tree-lined boulevards and a European feel.

Difficulty rating: Easy, entirely on accessible sidewalks.

Distance: 4 miles.

Estimated time: 2 hours.

Services: A number of restaurants and restrooms along the route. The Best Western, where the walk can start, also has a reasonably priced cafeteria-style restaurant, plus restrooms.

Restrictions: Dogs must be leashed and droppings picked up.

For more information: Contact the St. Louis Convention and Visitors Commission.

Getting started: This walk has two start options, one for those coming by car and another for those coming by MetroLink.

If you have driven to the Central West End, it will be easier to park your car if you start this walk at the Best Western Inn at the Park, 4630 Lindell Boulevard. Take Interstate 64/40 to the Kingshighway exit and go north to Lindell. Turn right on Lindell. The Best Western will be about a block down on your right. Park in its lot.

If you are taking the MetroLink, get off at the Central West End MetroLink station. The walk starts just outside the station at Children's Place in the hospital complex. If you have taken the MetroLink, turn to page 145, where your directions begin.

Public transportation: The MetroLink stops in the Central West End at Children's Place, where this walk can begin. Bi-State Transit Bus 18 stops within one block of the Best Western, the other start option.

Overview: The Central West End already was an established, elegant neighborhood when the 1904 World's Fair opened. The homes within limited-access streets known as "private places" date back to the late 1880s (see page 124).

The area offered wealthy St. Louisans not only open green spaces, but also refuge from the city. Most of St. Louis's movers and shakers lived here. In his history of St. Louis, James Neal Primm notes that "For at least three decades after 1900, the city's economic power, wealth, and social elite were concentrated within a half-dozen blocks of Lindell and Kingshighway."

Then, as now, an array of shops and restaurants and ornate lampposts could be found along Euclid Avenue and the nearby side streets. What you see today, however, is

Central West End

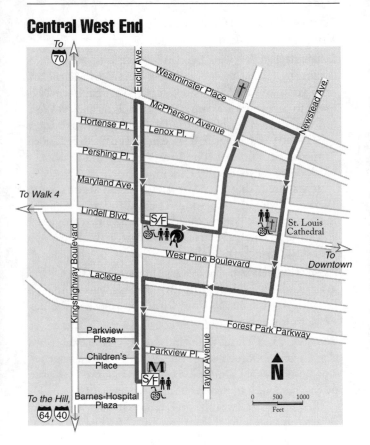

reclaimed beauty and usefulness. After World War II, the Central West End, like so many urban areas nationwide, had become blighted. Today, this neighborhood once again is vital and captivating.

Restored and well-maintained homes, trendy outdoor cafes, and one-of-a-kind shops lure people to the Central West End, making it one of the premier spots in which to walk and people watch. On a balmy weekend morning, when you are hunting for outdoor seating and a brunch menu, you will wish people found this area less alluring.

The walk

These directions start from the Best Western Inn at the Park. If you want to start this walk at the MetroLink Central West End station, turn to page 145.

➤As you leave the parking lot at the Best Western, turn right on Lindell Boulevard and walk one block to Taylor Avenue. Note the stone mansion coming up on your right as you approach Taylor. At the turn of the century, fine homes like this once lined Lindell all the way east to Grand Boulevard. This building, now the home of the archbishop of the Catholic Diocese of St. Louis, is among the street's few remaining mansions.

➤Cross Taylor. Turn left and cross Lindell. The sidewalks along these and other residential streets may have some bumps and uneven areas, but none large enough to impede a stroller or wheelchair.

This area of apartments has several lovely brownstones and ornate, decorative stonework. As you walk north on Taylor, look off to your left. These homes are not as distinguished as those you will see later, but they are lovely nonetheless.

➤At Westminster Place, turn right. The church you see across the street on the northwest corner is the Second Presbyterian Church, built in 1900. Theodore Link, the man who designed Union Station, designed this Richardsonian Romanesque Revival building and the building directly across the street, which was built in 1908 for the Wednesday Club, a women's organization.

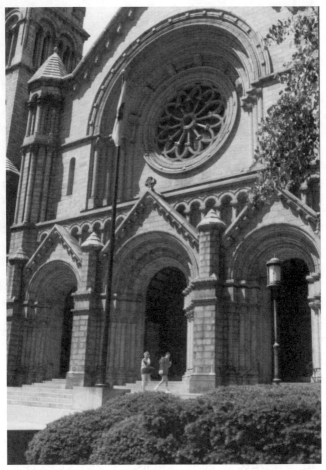

The Cathedral Basilica of Saint Louis anchors the eastern edge of the Central West End.

of interest

The Cathedral Basilica of Saint Louis

With its green-tiled dome, distinctive roof line, and two imposing towers, the cathedral is a noticeable and beloved structure in the St. Louis skyline. This imposing gray granite Romanesque church was begun in 1907 and completed in 1914. While the building itself is striking, it is the cathedral's mosaics that make it world famous.

Within its Byzantine interior, 83,000 square feet of mosaic art—almost two acres—covers the three domes, soffits, and arches. It is the single largest collection of mosaics in one building in the world. The mosaics in the vestibule and main church contain more than 41.5 million pieces of tesserae in more than eight thousand shades of color. The gleam of the gold leaf will take your breath away.

These sparkling representations capture angels, religious symbolism, the Creation, the lives of the saints, and some history of the church in St. Louis. Twenty artists contributed to this endeavor, which took seventy-five years to completely install.

As a testament to the church's significance among Roman Catholic churches, Rome deemed the cathedral a basilica in 1997. The New Cathedral now shares that distinction with the Old Cathedral.

The cathedral is open daily and welcomes visitors, so feel free to enter. You may want to start by sitting in a back pew and letting the grandeur wash over you before deciding which area of this massive church you wish to explore first.

The Mosaics Museum is on the lower level. Here you will also find the crypt of John Cardinal Glennon who started construction on the cathedral.

Volunteer guides and docents provide tours and explain the mosaics. Contact the cathedral for tour information or for a schedule of activities.

You are now entering Westminster Place. Begun in 1892, it is one of this area's most elegant and architecturally interesting private places. Many of the era's important architects designed at least one home here; they squeezed great architectural interest and diversity into a few blocks.

These homes sit squarely on their well-maintained lots. In the spring, the yards sparkle with blooms, rhododendron, and other flowering shrubs. The homes sport red-tiled roofs, stained glass, pillars, substantial stone steps, and roofs garnished with turrets, carvings, gables, and fireplace chimneys. Look for #4446. This red-brick four-story house was the family home of poet T.S. Eliot.

➤Go one block to Newstead Avenue and turn right. If you want to explore one more block of Westminster, do so now and return to this spot.

➤Follow Newstead back toward Lindell. The sidewalks along this stretch are a bit broken and uneven, so watch your footing. Newstead's homes, though not as grand as some others, are still charming.

➤After you cross Pershing Place, look for 325 North Newstead, which comes up on your right. Cathedral Tower once housed parochial schools for boys and girls. Today it houses young mothers and the elderly.

You are approaching the back of the Cathedral Basilica of Saint Louis. Locals call this Roman Catholic church the New Cathedral, to distinguish it from the Old Cathedral downtown. Be sure to take a moment and go inside. The accessible entrance can be found just off the rear parking lot.

➤When you leave the cathedral, cross Lindell and continue south on Newstead. Across the street at #12-14, you will find an old police station that has been revamped into office space. The tall, arched window replaced the doorway that once opened for the mounted police. Built in 1905, the Newstead District Police Station was active until 1960. The station has an intriguing secret. It is said that when kidnappers and their suitcases of ransom money were captured and brought to the station, one-half of the $600,000 disappeared. Some think the money may still be hidden within the building.

➤At Laclede Avenue, turn right. Two- and three-story brick homes line this quaint street. Some of the homes are still being reclaimed and restored.

➤At Euclid Avenue, turn left. You are heading into the hospital complex and toward the MetroLink station, which will be on your left, by a flower shop, just past Children's Place.

This area of tall buildings and bustle contains several health care facilities: Jewish Hospital founded in 1900 to care for indigent Jewish immigrants, and Barnes Hospital, founded in 1914, merged with Christian Hospital in 1996. The three now operate as BJC. You also will find Children's Hospital, the medical and dental schools for both St. Louis University and Washington University, the St. Louis College of Pharmacy, the Jewish Hospital School of Nursing, and the Central Institute for the Deaf. If you are feeling ill, you have come to the right place.

➤At Children's Place, cross to the other side of Euclid.

Please note: The directions for those beginning this walk at the MetroLink station start here.

Your walk north along Euclid will take you to the shops and restaurants that have made this street so delightful. The Majestic Restaurant at the corners of Euclid and Laclede is a popular spot, serving generous portions from breakfast through dinner. Elsewhere you will find dishes from India, China, and the Mideast, pizza, pasta, health foods, bagels, deli subs, and ice cream. Get ready to nosh your way along Euclid to McPherson Avenue and back—more than a mile of edible temptation.

➤At Hortense Place you may want to leave Euclid and explore this block-long private place of large, elegant homes.

➤As you approach the corner of Euclid and McPherson, you enter another popular shopping and dining area. Left Bank Books, a friendly and jam-packed bookstore, is on the southwest corner in a turn-of-the-century building. Across the street to the north is Balaban's cafe and restaurant, offering delightful provisions in a trendy atmosphere. Across the street to your right is Rothchild's Antiques. Step inside even if you cannot think of a thing you need. You are sure to spot other shops and restaurants that catch your attention.

➤At McPherson, turn right and cross Euclid. You now will head back on the other side of Euclid. Before you do, walk east along McPherson for a few feet until you come to Karl Bissinger's French Confections. Bissinger's has made French candies in this location since 1927. The decor is original, and the three-hundred-year-old candy recipes produce heavenly treats.

➤Return to Euclid and go to your left. The first street on your left is Lenox Place; like Hortense, this is another private place. Walk the block in and back if you want to view these homes.

➤Continue another block to Pershing Place. If you have any interest in Beat generation writer William Burroughs, turn left on Pershing and look for # 4664, a place where he once lived.

➤Return to Euclid and continue south to Lindell. The Women's Club Building on the corner at 4600 Lindell was built to host international visitors during the World's Fair. It is now a private club.

➤Cross Lindell, turn left, and return to the Inn at the Park and the end of this walk. If you are continuing to the MetroLink start of this walk, turn to page 141 for the remaining directions.

Do you have some walking energy left? From the Central West End MetroLink station, you can take either the Shuttle Bug or the MetroLink to Forest Park and Walk 4. The Forest Park MetroLink station is one block north of the Jefferson Memorial Building, the walk's start. You can also catch the Shuttle Bug to Forest Park from the east side of the cathedral. The shuttle stops at the Jefferson Memorial Building or at one of five other park attractions that are along the route of Walk 4.

walk 14
The Hill

General location: You will find the Hill on the city's south-west side, just south of Forest Park.

Special attractions: Fantastic Italian food, fun Italian grocery stores, a well-tended and charming neighborhood.

Difficulty rating: Easy, flat, entirely on sidewalks.

Distance: 1 mile.

Estimated time: 30 minutes.

Services: Restaurants, restrooms only in places of business and Berra Park.

Restrictions: Most of the restaurants and all of the stores are closed on Sunday. Some of the restaurants are wheelchair accessible.

For more information: Contact the St. Louis Convention and Visitors Commission.

The Hill

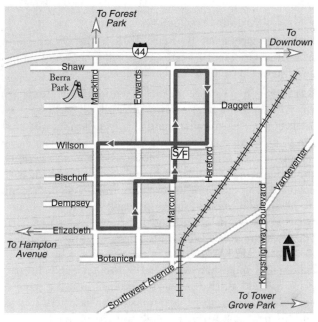

Getting started: This walk starts at the front of St. Ambrose's Church, which is at the corner of Wilson and Marconi avenues, in the heart of the Hill. Interstate 44 cuts through the northern section of this neighborhood. At Hampton Avenue take I-44 Exit 286 and go south one short block to Wilson. Turn left on Wilson and go about six blocks to Marconi. You will see the church on your right.

Kingshighway Boulevard, the Hill's eastern boundary line, is a major north-south street. Take I-44, Exit 287. Then take Kingshighway south to Southwest Avenue and turn right. Take Southwest to Marconi, the first street that comes up on the right. Turn right and take Marconi four blocks to

Wilson. Look for a place to park along the side streets near the church. Depending on the day and time when you come to the Hill, parking may be scarce.

Public transportation: Bi-State Transit Bus 99 stops on Macklind. Contact Bi-State to confirm other routes, stops, and times.

Overview: When you see the green, white, and red fireplugs, you will know you have entered the Hill. The area was first settled by northern Italians in the early 1900s; they had left the Illinois coal fields to mine clay for St. Louis's booming terra cotta and fire-brick businesses. For almost a century, the Hill has maintained its ethnic flavor, and even today an estimated 75 percent of its residents are of Italian descent.

This area of modest but impeccably maintained homes was the boyhood neighborhood of baseball greats Yogi Berra and Joe Garagiola. But the area has not always looked so tidy. Post World War II flight to the suburbs brought vacant houses and urban decay. In the 1960s, a triple threat—plans to build a drive-in theater, interest in using the old, abandoned clay mines as a dumpsite for industrial wastes, and Interstate 44 cutting through and separating the neighborhood—sparked strong interest in preservation and restoration.

The community fought off two of the threats. However, the interstate was built, but so were a walkway and bridges to reconnect the divided neighborhood. Today the Hill stands as a strong example of the power of community spirit in the efforts of urban renewal.

The walk

This walk starts at the front of St. Ambrose Catholic Church—the cultural, community, and spiritual center of the Hill. Go to the green sign that announces, "Welcome to the

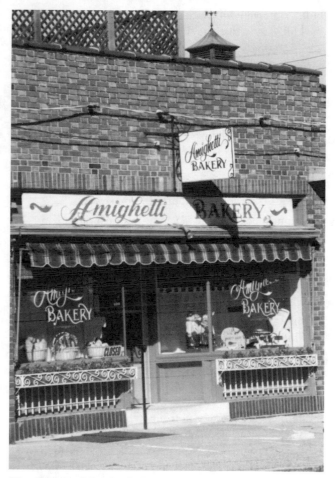

The windows of Amighetti's Bakery are likely to lure anyone with a sweet tooth inside.

Hill." Here you will find a map and business directory of the Hill. As you face the sign, Wilson Avenue is to your left.

➤Cross Wilson and start north on Marconi. To your right is Amighetti's, a delicious mixture of bakery, restaurant, and ice cream shop. This eatery is famous throughout the city for its submarine sandwiches.

Milo's Bocce Garden is across the street and to your left. Bocce, a form of lawn bowling, is popular on the Hill. This older looking block contains two-story homes and businesses.

➤ At the next corner, Daggett Avenue and Marconi, you will spot DiGregorio's Imported Food store.

➤Go one block to Shaw Avenue and turn right. Kitty corner and across the street is the up-scale restaurant Giovanni's on the Hill. Across the street is the Italian grocery Viviano's and Sons. Even if you are not interested in shopping for Italian ingredients, pop in just to inhale the aromas and to peek at the store's many intriguing items.

➤Follow Shaw to Hereford Street and turn right.

This part of this old, but well-maintained, working-class neighborhood has small, often narrow, houses. Bricked or sided, bungalows or two-stories, most of the homes have small flower gardens and manicured lawns. Now and then you will spot a grotto devoted to the Blessed Mother or a resident out scrubbing the front steps.

At the corner of Daggett and Hereford, you will find Fabio's Pasta and Grill. Note its lovely leaded-glass and wood door. Across the street, the homes are especially tiny, with narrow fronts and few windows.

➤Go one more block to Wilson and turn right.

Dominic's Restaurant is on the corner, and St. Ambrose School is across the street. Farther down on your side of the street, you will walk past Amighetti's Bakery window. Stop and peek in. If you feel the urge to sample a cannoli, give in!

Cross Marconi and continue west on Wilson. The drivers have the stop signs, but cross with care.

This entirely residential block repeats the urban, neighborhood feel. Wood or wrought-iron fences, and small front yards, many with yard ornaments, give this street a tended look.

➤Cross Edwards Street and continue on Wilson.

Zia's Restaurant is on the corner. This area of the Hill is a little younger, built up as the immigrants became more established. The houses are larger and not as modest.

➤At Macklind Avenue and Wilson, turn left and cross Wilson. The traffic on Wilson does not have a stop sign. On your left is the Sacred Heart Villa school.

➤Cross Bischoff Avenue, a four-way stop. Across the street, on the corner, is Momma Toscano's Ravioli. In this area, the bungalows look more substantial.

➤At Elizabeth, turn left.

➤At Edwards, turn left. Augusti's Restaurant is across the street and on the corner.

As soon as you make the turn onto Edwards, the street instantly feels more urban. Perhaps it is the absence of trees and grass or the presence of more utility wires and poles that gives this block an older, urban ambiance.

➤Go to Bischoff and Edwards. The Oldani Brothers Sausage Company is on your left, offering salami, choice cuts of meats and party trays, and Italian specialties. Across the street is Mama Campisi's.

➤Turn right and cross Edwards at Bischoff.

➤Go one block to Marconi.

of interest

Pasta pleasures

If you say you are "going to The Hill," folks naturally assume you are hungry for Italian food—spaghetti in a rich marinara sauce, crisp salads dressed with tangy vinegar and oil house dressings, hearty lasagna, flavorful salami and prosciutto, imported Italian cheeses, fresh-baked bread, aromatic basil and oregano, and cannoli stuffed with sweetened ricotta. And let's not forget toasted ravioli, which was created in a Hill restaurant. These meat-filled pasta pillows are rolled in bread crumbs, deep fried and then smothered in meat sauce.

You will find a restaurant on almost every corner—one is sure to suit your palate, budget, and attire. If you want a little candlelight and atmosphere, try the more upscale, Northern Italian food at Giovanni's or Dominic's, where the waiters sport tuxedos. Want food served in a mom-and-pop atmosphere? Then scout out Zia's or Mama Campisi's, which is one of the few Hill restaurants open on Sundays. For hearty sandwiches and homemade ice cream, you can't beat Amighetti's—a combination of bakery, sub shop, outdoor garden and gelateria.

One of the city's most popular Italian restaurants, Cunetto House of Pasta, is just to the south on Southwest Avenue. Come hungry—the portions are generous.

Want some freshly made sausage and mozzarella cheese for your own Italian dinner? Then pop into John Viviano and Sons, a grocery replete with everything an Italian cook needs—from fresh pasta to a deep and decorative lasagna pan. The aroma alone will have you salivating!

➤Cross Marconi. Turn left and cross Bischoff. You will pass Vitale's Bakery—offering Italian bread, homemade pasta, and pizza shells—and next door to that is Gian-Peppe's Restaurant.

➤Return to the front of St. Ambrose's Church and the end of this walk. If any of the stores or restaurants intrigued you during this walk, check out the green Welcome sign to find your way back to these establishments.

Walk 15

The MetroLink Walk

General location: Along the city's light-rail system, from Lambert International Airport on the west to Laclede's Landing and the Mississippi River on the east.

Special attractions: Most all the sights worth seeing within the core of St. Louis.

Difficulty rating: Most of the walking options are easy and on sidewalks. If you are pushing a stroller or using a wheelchair, be sure to read through the complete walk directions, so you can anticipate places where the path may have steps or curbs.

Distance: Anywhere from 1 to 30 miles.

Estimated time: From 30 minutes to all day.

Services: Many restaurants, restrooms, and shops, depending on where you decide to walk.

The MetroLink Walk

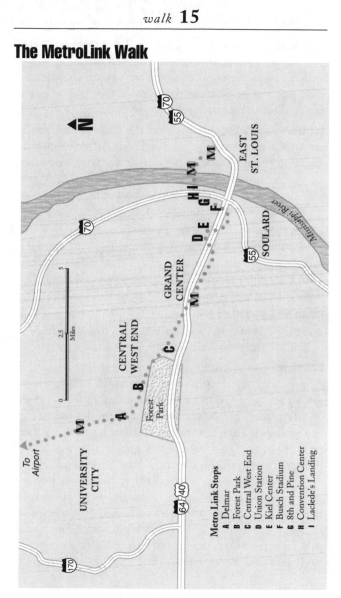

Metro Link Stops

A Delmar
B Forest Park
C Central West End
D Union Station
E Kiel Center
F Busch Stadium
G 8th and Pine
H Convention Center
I Laclede's Landing

Restrictions: On the MetroLink or Bi-State Transit buses, you cannot smoke, eat, drink, litter, or use audio players without an earphone. You cannot travel with animals other than guide dogs. Seats at the front of the train or bus are reserved for the elderly and those with disabilities.

For more information: Glance over the walks in this book to see which suit your time and interests. If you want more specific information about travel times, fares, and routes along the MetroLink or bus lines, contact Bi-State Transit. Call the museums or attractions found in the various walks for information about their times, fees, and exhibits.

Getting started: You can start a walk at any one of the sixteen MetroLink stops found in St. Louis or from the two found just across the Mississippi River in Illinois. As you can see from the map, you are only a quick Metro ride away from more than half the walks in this book.

Public transportation: For these walks, public transportation is at the heart of getting where you want to walk. Check the individual walks for train and bus information.

Overview: If you have time to kill at Lambert International Airport, are staying at a downtown hotel, simply want to ditch your car, or want to see a great deal of St. Louis in a few days, then get on the MetroLink and let the ride get you walking. This new transportation network connects eighteen MetroLink stations along an eighteen-mile track that stretches from the airport to East St. Louis, Illinois.

The system runs more than thirty electrically powered vehicles from about 5 a.m. to 1 a.m. and offers an inexpensive, fast, and efficient way to travel. Eight of the MetroLink stations have a total of 2,500 free "Park-n-Ride" spaces, while parking at the other stations can be found on the street or in paid lots. Those stations that offer free parking have a parking symbol noted on the map. Bicycles also are permitted on the trains.

The MetroLink runs on the honor system. You buy a ticket at one of the vending machines located in each station or from one of more than two hundred area businesses that sell transit passes and tickets. These businesses include drugstores, groceries, and banks. Tickets can also be purchased at the MetroRide Store, just inside the Seventh and Washington streets entrance of downtown's St. Louis Centre. No tickets are sold on the trains.

Passengers must carry a valid ticket or pass on the train and may be asked to show proof of payment to an inspector. Passengers caught without a ticket may pay a substantial fine and must make a court appearance.

You can ride free between Union Station and Laclede's Landing every Monday through Friday between 10 a.m. and 3 p.m. The all-day pass, however, is a real bargain. For three dollars passengers have an unlimited number of rides on the MetroLink and buses.

MetroLink stations are fully accessible. They include elevators to and from those train platforms not level with the street and ramps.

The walk

Your ride-and-walk excursion can start anywhere along the MetroLink line. However, these directions assume you are starting at Lambert International Airport, the rail's western point. No Metro station is more than thirty minutes away from Lambert. So, if you are waiting a few hours for a flight, you may be able to squeeze in a walk. Remember, the times listed with each walk estimate only the walking time. Sightseeing is extra.

➤You will find a MetroLink train at the eastern end of the terminal on the main level. Go past the ticket counters and follow the signs for the MetroLink station, which is outdoors. Your walk is now just a few minutes away. The station at Delmar is the first place where you can get off and find a walk.

Delmar Stop
Walk 12, University City

➤At Delmar, exit the train and follow the sidewalk to the street.

➤Go to your right and walk along Delmar Boulevard for about four blocks. Just past Skinker Boulevard, at the city limits of St. Louis and University City, you will connect with the walking route for Walk 12. Turn to page 135 and your directions in the middle of the page.

Forest Park Stop
Walk 4, Park Tour

➤When you leave the station walk about one block along DeBaliviere Boulevard toward Forest Park.

➤You will cross Forest Park Parkway and then Lindell Boulevard. The walk begins on page 52 in front of the Jefferson Memorial Building.

Walk 5, St. Louis Zoo

➤When you exit the station, take the Shuttle Bug, the red mini-bus with the black spots. The Bug will drop you off at the entrance to the zoo. The walk starts on page 68.

Central West End Stop
Walk 6, Missouri Botanical Garden

➤At the MetroLink Station, transfer to Bus 13, which will take you to the entrance of the gardens and the walk's start.

Walk 7, Tower Grove Park, and Walk 8, Grand South Grand

➤At the MetroLink Station, transfer to Bus 95. Get off at Tower Grove Park at the corner of Kingshighway Boulevard and Arsenal Street. Walk into the park. Your walk starts a few blocks away, just north of the traffic circle by the park's Magnolia Street entrance. Turn to page 94 for your directions.

➤Walk 8 starts just outside the park's Grand Street Entrance on its east side. You can intersect with the start of that walk while following the directions for Walk 7. If you want to go directly to Walk 8, follow Arsenal along the park until you reach Grand Boulevard, which is 1.4 miles to the east. Turn to page 100 for your directions.

Walk 13, Central West End

➤When you exit the Metro, you are at one of the two start points for this walk.

➤Cross Euclid Street and turn to page 145 for your directions.

Grand Station Stop

No walks start near the MetroLink's Grand Station. However, Bus 70, which stops here, will take you north on Grand to the city's arts and entertainment district. Known as Grand Center, this restored eight-block-square area includes many cultural offerings. The most well-known are Powell Hall, home to the St. Louis Symphony, the second oldest symphony orchestra in the country. The Fabulous Fox Theatre, a restored 1929 movie palace, hosts touring entertainment, and the Black Repertory Company performs in the Grandel Square Theatre.

Union Station Stop
Walk 3, City Sights

➤When you leave the train, take the stairs or elevator up to street level. You are now in the back of Union Station. The walk begins in front of the station at the corners of Market and 20th streets.

➤To get to the start, walk into Union Station and follow the thoroughfare past the shops.

➤When you reach the fountain by the information booth, turn left and follow the shop-lined corridor to the exit at 20th Street.

➤Turn right and go to corner. Turn to page 40 for your directions.

Kiel Center Stop
Walk 3, City Sights

➤Walk 3 passes in front of Kiel Auditorium. So when you leave the station, walk toward Market Street and turn to page 50 for the tail end of Walk 3. When you reach the walk's end, turn to page 40 to start the walk.

Whether you exit at this station or not, be sure to look for a pink and tan building that is near the station and visible from the train windows. This 1920s warehouse has wonderful architectural details, such as obelisks and windows, and some fanciful ones, such as angels and eagles. It is all a trompe l'oeil—painted on, yet so real.

Busch Stadium Stop
Walk 3, City Sights

➤When you are at street level, you will be on the southwest side of Busch Stadium.

➤Cross Seventh Street.

of interest

Travel tips

These tips will help make your MetroLink trip more enjoyable:

➤ Know which direction you want to go. East? West? Then get on the correct platform. If you get on a train going the wrong way, get out at the next stop and cross over to the correct platform.

➤ Avoid buying your tickets at night from station vending machines. If you know you will be using public transportation throughout the day or for several days, buy a one-day, three-day, or week pass.

➤ If you are traveling alone in off hours, stand near others on the platform.

➤ If you hear a train approaching, do not race to the platform. Another train will come soon. Trains run about every 10 to 15 minutes, and about every 30 minutes on weekends before 7:30 a.m. and after about 10 p.m. No trains run from about midnight to 5 a.m.

➤Turn to page 48 for the rest of the walk directions, which will have you going left alongside the stadium's west side.

Walk 7, Tower Grove Park, and Walk 8, Grand South Grand

➤Take Bus 21, which stops at Busch Stadium, to the corner of Arsenal Street and Grand Boulevard. For Walk 8, turn to page 100 and pick up the directions as they cross Arsenal near the start of Walk 8.

You can connect with Walk 7 at the park's east Grand Street entrance. After you enter the gates, turn to page 96 to pick up the walk's trail.

Walk 6, Missouri Botanical Garden

►Take Bus 99, which stops at the gardens. Turn to page 80 for your directions.

Walk 9, Soulard

►Take Bus 99, which stops at Busch Stadium, and ask the driver to let you off at Soulard Market. The walk starts at the market's entrance. Turn to page 106 for the directions.

Walk 11, Lafayette Street

►Take Bus 99, which stops at Busch Stadium, and ask the driver to let you off at the corner of Lafayette and Mississippi Avenues. Walk to the park. Walk 11 circles Lafayette Park, so turn to page 121 for the commentary.

8th and Pine Stop

Walk 3, City Sights

►When you come up to street level, walk south one block toward Chestnut. To get your bearings, the Arch will be on your left as you walk toward Chestnut. Turn to page 48 and the point where you intersect the walk at Chestnut and 7th.

Buses 21 and 99 also stop here and can take you to walks 7, 8, 9, and 11. You can find the bus comments for these walks just above at Busch Stadium Stop.

Convention Center Station

Walk 3, City Sights

►When you reach street level, you will be on Washington Street and the path for Walk 3. Turn to page 45 and the directions that start from this point.

Laclede's Landing Station

Walk 1, Jefferson National Expansion Memorial; Walk 2, Laclede's Landing; and Walk 3, City Sights

➤When you take the elevator or steps down from the train platform, you will be on Second Street at the corner of Washington Avenue. Walk 2 starts here. Turn to page 34 for your directions.

➤Walk 1 starts across the street at one of the park entrances. Turn to page 25 for your directions.

➤Walk 3 passes by here on Washington. Turn to page 45 and the directions that pass this point.

walk 16
Bellefontaine Cemetery

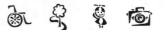

General location: North of Interstate 70 in the city's northeast section.

Special attractions: Ornate monuments and mausoleums, park setting and lush landscaping, historic gravesites of city's most notable people.

Difficulty rating: Easy, flat, entirely on paved roadways.

Distance: 3.5 miles.

Estimated time: 2 hours.

Services: Restrooms and water available only at the main entrance. The restrooms are wheelchair-accessible, but the building has steps leading to its entrance.

Restrictions: Although this is a private cemetery, visitors are invited to come and appreciate the beautiful grounds and the rich history captured here. However, please remember that the grounds are a place for serenity and reflection.

The cemetery is open daily from 8 a.m. to 5 p.m., and its gates are locked promptly at 5 p.m. If you start your walk in the afternoon, be sure to allow enough time, so that you and your car are not caught inside. The cemetery staff asks that children be accompanied by adults and that no one picnic or bring alcohol onto the grounds.

For more information: Contact Bellefontaine Cemetery.

Getting started: You can reach this cemetery by taking Interstate 70 to the West Florissant Exit 245B. Then go north on West Florissant Avenue for about half a mile. The cemetery entrance will be on your right. Turn right, park near the main office, and stop in to request a free map. It includes a key to the resting places of the more famous inhabitants. Other informative materials on the cemetery and its history are on sale, should you wish to learn more.

Public transportation: Bi-State Transit Bus 95 stops on West Florissant near both the Bellefontaine and Calvary Cemeteries' entrances. Contact Bi-State for information on schedules and fares.

Overview: Most early St. Louisans were first buried on the city's western borders along what is now Jefferson Avenue. Because the living of the ever-expanding city soon needed more room, the old cemeteries had to be relocated. In March 1849, a committee of prominent citizens established a large, private, nonsectarian cemetery five miles outside the city limits to the northwest. They named it Bellefontaine because one of the nearby roads led to Fort Bellefontaine, which had been deactivated in 1826. The first 137-acre tract purchased for the cemetery had once been farmed by the Hempstead family, and the family's private burial plot was incorporated into the new cemetery.

Bellefontaine Cemetery

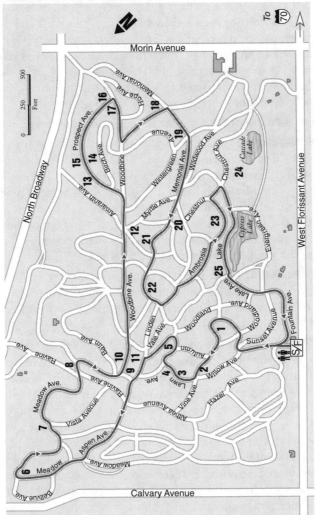

Memorial Markers

1	Thomas Hart Benton	13	David Rowland Francis
2	Virginia L. Miner	14	Charlotte Dickson Wainwright
3	Robert Campbell	15	Lemp Mausoleum
4	Joseph Charless/Taylor Blow	16	George Warren Brown
5	James Eads	17	A.D. Brown
6	William Clark	18	James S. McDonnell
7	Stephen Hempstead/Manuel Lisa	19	Herman Luyties
8	Buell/Mason Family	20	Chris Von der Ahe
9	Susan Elizabeth Blow	21	Sara Teasdale
10	Isaiah Sellers	22	John R. O'Fallon
11	Busch Mausoleum	23	George Vest
12	Laumeier Family	24	Severson Family
		25	William S. Burroughs

Bellefontaine was established just in time, because cholera struck with deadly force that June. During one week in July, more than seven hundred people died, the majority of them small children and recent immigrants. By August, St. Louis had lost one-tenth of its citizens.

The resting place of the city's cholera victims looks nothing like the park you will walk and where more than 86,000 people now are buried. The fourteen miles of winding paths, manmade lakes, and the landscaping of the eventual 310 acres were developed over time by Almerin Hotchkiss, who left his job with a cemetery in Brooklyn, New York, to become superintendent of Bellefontaine. Hotchkiss nurtured these lush, peaceful grounds for forty-six years. His son Frank assumed the job for the next twenty.

Mike Tiemann, the current superintendent, notes that Bellefontaine is an excellent example of a cemetery that grew out of the garden-as-cemetery movement. In the 1830s, New England's bleak graveyards gave way to beautifully landscaped parks, the precursors to this country's many city parks. So, before St. Louisans ambled through Forest Park on Sunday afternoons, they strolled in Bellefontaine and neighboring Calvary Cemetery.

Back in the late 1800s, those who walked by these imposing mausoleums, towering obelisks, and life-size statues of angels and mortals saw the names of people they knew, people who had helped to build the city and tame the West. Today this marble and granite metropolis silently utters the history of a young country and of one of its oldest cities.

The walk

Bellefontaine is a labyrinth of winding roadways that at times seem to coil around each other. You may feel a little like Alice in Wonderland as she tried to decipher directions from the Cheshire Cat. To help you stay on the described path, we have included reference points, such as the names on nearby monuments or descriptions of statues, to help you pick the right road. We also encourage you to meander among these striking monuments, described by one sculptor as "magical stone forests." But be sure to return to the point where you left the roadway.

➤Start at the cemetery office and go down Willow Avenue.

➤Turn right at Laurel Avenue. The Pocock plot is to your right.

➤Stay on Laurel. Do not take Sunset Avenue, which will come up on your right just as you turn onto Laurel.

➤Cross the Woodland Avenue intersection. Laurel will curve to the left. If you pass the tall Gay family monument with its draped urn on your left, you will know you are on the right road.

Look off to your left and search for the polished red granite obelisk. This is the tomb of Thomas Hart Benton, who became a U.S. senator when Missouri entered the Union in 1821.

➤When you leave the Benton grave, continue to the T intersection.

➤Turn right on Woodland, which will soon become Vine Avenue at the intersection of Vine and Autumn Avenues.

➤Continue straight on Vine. The smaller Minor obelisk will be on your left. Virginia L. Minor was a suffragist and a lawyer who sued the local election commissioners when they denied her the right to vote. She lost on appeal to the U.S. Supreme Court. After the Minor grave, Willow Avenue comes up on your left and Lawn Avenue on your right.

➤Follow Lawn to your right. The large Peper family monument is to your right as you make the turn onto Lawn. Low stone fencing, accented with large urns, encircles the gray granite obelisk of Robert Campbell, who made his fortune in fur trading. His home at Fifteenth and Locust is furnished in period furniture and is open to the public.

➤Shortly after Campbell, you will come to a T intersection. To your left and slightly in from the road is the marker for Joseph Charless and the Blow family. Charless established the first newspaper west of the Mississippi. Taylor Blow is remembered as the man who owned and then freed the slave Dred Scott.

➤At the T intersection, go to your right. You will see the street names of Lawn and Autumn Avenues. Autumn points to your right, which is the way you are going. On your right, you will see an obelisk with a cross, which marks the plot of the Pettus family.

➤Follow the road as it curves left. The signpost says you have entered Memory Avenue. Immediately on the left, you will see the carved stone casket with the name Eads at its base. Engineer James Eads designed the first steel construction bridge to span the Mississippi River and the iron-clad gunboats that helped the Union win the Civil War.

➤Immediately after passing the Eads plot, you will come to a four-corner intersection and go left. The Milburn family plot is directly to your right as you make this turn.

➤At the next intersection, you will see up ahead the back of the elaborate, pink granite mausoleum of Adolphus Busch. Later you will pass the front of this ornate structure.

➤Turn left on Vale at this intersection. The road signs indicate you are at the crossroad of Vale and Woodland.

➤At the next intersection, you will see the Snow family markers low to the ground and directly in front of you. The street sign says Lawn, and you will go to your right.

➤Within a few feet, the road becomes a Y intersection. You will take the left arm of the Y. The street sign says Aspen and points to your left. You will know you are on the right path when immediately on the left you see a wrought-iron fenced enclosure for Scott.

➤Take Aspen straight ahead for a few blocks.

➤Where Aspen intersects with Meadow Avenue, head right on Meadow. The street sign may be a bit crooked. You will know you made the correct choice if the Knittel-Bierman family monument is to your left.

➤Continue on Meadow.

➤At the Y intersection of Bellvue Avenue and Meadow, continue on Meadow.

➤At the T intersection, turn right. Immediately on your right, you will see a large, gray obelisk surrounded by several smaller memorials. This is the burial site of General William Clark, leader of the exploration of the Louisiana Purchase. The inscription on the obelisk is a quote from Deuteronomy: "Behold the Lord thy God has set the land before thee: Go up and possess it."

Step into the Clark circle and read the markers and Clark's history. The tombstone of Clark's oldest son speaks of the regard Clark felt for his comrade Meriwether Lewis. In 1809, the year Lewis died, Clark's son, Meriwether Lewis Clark, was born. When you return to the road, turn to your right. You will soon pass the cemetery's oldest graves.

➤Follow Meadow, always keeping to the left when other roads intersect. Shortly after you pass Elm Avenue on your right, look to your left along Meadow for the Lisa and Hempstead obelisks. They will be more obvious after you pass the Winkelmeyer plots. Lisa's monument is behind the Uhrig obelisk, and behind Lisa is Hempstead.

These are the cemetery's oldest graves. Stephen Hempstead served in the Revolutionary War. Manuel Lisa, a bold and powerful fur trader, married Hempstead's daughter Mary. She is thought to be the first white woman to enter the Indian territory of the upper Missouri River.

➤Continue on Meadow, which will curve to the right. If you look to your left, you can look down on the rail yards and sense the cemetery's bluff location. This is one of the few areas in the cemetery where you still see an open expanse of land. After you pass the three hillside crypts, you will go downhill slightly.

➤At the four-corner intersection, cross Ravine Avenue.

➤Take the first right after crossing Ravine; this is Lawn. Note the Buell memorial to the left. Major General Don Carlos Buell, his wife, Margaret Hunter Mason Buell, and her first husband, Brigadier General Richard B. Mason, are buried on the same lot. The man who designed Mason's tomb also designed the sarcophagus of George and Martha Washington.

➤Pass Balm Avenue on your left.

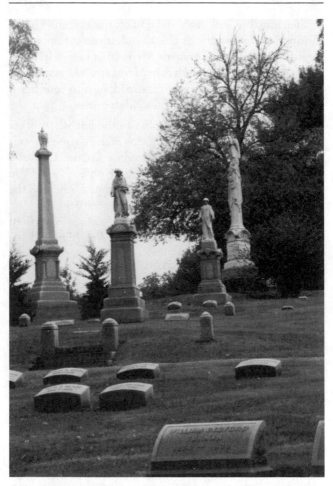

More than memorials, the markers at Bellefontaine Cemetery are works of art.

➤Take the next left, which is Woodbine Avenue. Follow Woodbine for several blocks and pass three notable grave sites. First on your right will be the tomb of Henry T. Blow and his daughter Susan Elizabeth Blow. She started the country's first public kindergarten in St. Louis in 1873.

Across the road from the Busch mausoleum, find the tombstone with the carving of a riverboat captain. Captain Isaiah Sellers, a famous riverboat man, navigated the Mississippi for forty years. He wrote under the pseudonym Mark Twain, the name Samuel Clemens later adopted as his own.

The Busch mausoleum—perhaps the cemetery's most ornate—holds the remains of Adolphus Busch and Lilly Anheuser Busch. Lilly's father, Eberhard Anheuser, founded the famous brewery and is buried in a simpler grave behind the mausoleum.

➤Continue east on Woodbine. On your right, at the intersection of Myrtle Avenue and Woodbine, you will see the family plot of the Laumeiers, the family that established the Laumeier Sculpture Park—the site of Walk 20. This dramatic family plot includes pieces resembling chess rooks. Directly in front is a hitching post, one of the few remaining in the cemetery.

➤At Woodbine and Prospect, go left on Prospect. You will spot Prospect in part because on your right you will see the Dozier monument with its detailed palm leaf carved into granite.

Once on Prospect, look to your left for the shrouded and mournful specter guarding the tomb of David Rowland Francis, a former St. Louis mayor, Missouri governor, U.S. Secretary of the Interior under President Cleveland, and U.S. ambassador to Imperial Russia during the Communist overthrow. Francis also was president of the St. Louis World's Fair. Francis Field at Washington University, his alma mater, is named for him.

To your right, directly across from the David Francis tomb, is the Hills obelisk, the tallest in St. Louis and one of the tallest in America. Its total weight is more than 100 tons.

Also on your right is the Wainwright tomb. Designed by famed architect Louis Sullivan, this limestone cube with its rounded roof is on the National Register of Historic Places. Millionaire Ellis Wainwright had it built for his young wife, Charlotte Dickson Wainwright.

Directly across from Wainwright is the Lemp family tomb, the cemetery's largest mausoleum. Wealthy brewers, the Lemps were among the city's notable families. You will see their mansion on Walk 10. Stand in front of the mausoleum and catch the light as it streams through the golden window glass.

You might notice that this area with its rows of elegant mausoleums looks like a neighborhood of miniature mansions.

➤At the T intersection, go right on Woodbine. Note the hexagonal mausoleum of shoe manufacturer George Warren Brown on your right and the circular mausoleum to brother A. D. Brown on the left.

On your right as you walk along Woodbine, you will pass several mausoleums in a row: the classic Greek temple of the Millikens; the tomb of the Spink family, publishers of baseball's *Sporting News*; and the Egyptian-style mausoleum of the Tate family.

➤Turn left at Walnut. Depending on when you walk, you may catch the aroma of baking bread from the nearby Wonder Bread factory.

➤Stop at the four-corner intersection of Walnut and Memorial and look to your left and a bit back for a large, rectangular bench bearing the name McDonnell. This is the tomb of James S. McDonnell, whose company was one of the largest manufacturers of jets, spacecraft, and missiles.

➤Turn right onto Memorial. At the next intersection, look to your right for the tomb with the "girl in the shadow box." While in Italy, Herman Luyties fell in love with a sculptor's model. He proposed; she declined. So he asked the sculptor to create this twelve-foot, several-ton likeness of the young beauty. Eventually the statue was moved to the family burial plot, and he rests forever at her feet.

➤Continue on Memorial. As you pass Myrtle, look to your left for the monument with the standing gentleman. Chris Von der Ahe was an early owner of the St. Louis Browns, the city's first baseball team. His tomb, bearing the correct year of his death, was erected while he lived.

Coming up on your right and back from the road is the grave of Sara Teasdale, the first person to win a Pulitzer Prize for poetry. Look for the large, gray triangular obelisk. If you walk toward it, you will find the Teasdale family plot directly to the left. Most likely flags or flowers decorate Sara's grave.

➤Continue on Memorial. Look for the large gray obelisk coming up on your left. This monument with a statue of a woman at its top, stands in the center of the O'Fallon family plot, the largest lot in the cemetery. Businessman John R. O'Fallon was a major benefactor of higher education in St. Louis.

➤Follow the road as it curves around the O'Fallon plot, which will stay to your left.

➤At the back side of the O'Fallon memorial, after you have circled almost halfway around it, you will come upon a three-forked intersection.

➤Take the right fork in the road, which you will soon see from the signs is Ambrosia Avenue.

➤Stay on Ambrosia. You will notice Cypress Lake to your right in the distance.

➤At the next intersection, with the Hoffman mausoleum that looks like an old church on your right, you will turn right.

➤Turn left on the road that comes up almost immediately to your left. As you make the left curve, the street marker says Hemlock. Now look to your left for a red, rough-cut boulder behind the Jackson memorial. The boulder marks the grave of U.S. Senator George Vest, who helped establish this country's national park system.

➤Continue on Hemlock.

➤Turn right at the intersection of Hemlock and Chestnut Avenue. The Corbitt memorial will be directly behind the Chestnut sign.

➤Stop for a moment at the intersection of Lake and Chestnut. To your left is Cascade Lake. Just before the lake is a narrow, eighteen-foot stone carved from Salisbury pink granite. You may wish to view the marker that sculptor William Severson created for his family plot. This upright stone, or stele, allows the sun of the winter and summer solstice to shine through its slits, forming a cross of light.

➤Turn right at the intersection of Chestnut and Lake and walk toward Cypress Lake.

➤You will walk along Lake Avenue to the lake's farthest tip.

➤Stop at the intersection of Lake and Vale. To your right is a gray granite obelisk for William S. Burroughs, the inventor of the mechanical adding machine—the precursor of the computer. Another Burroughs is also buried here—the beat-generation writer William S. Burroughs, who died in 1997. His unmarked grave is to the right as you face the obelisk.

➤Return to the corners of Lake and Vale.

➤Follow Lake uphill. The Burroughs plot will be behind you; the Rogers family plot with the girl statue will be on your right; the Diederich stone to your left.

➤Turn left at the top of the hill, where you face the marker for Mattie Morgan.

➤Stay on Lake until it merges into Fountain Avenue. You will be walking toward an angel standing in front of a cross.

➤Take Fountain back to the office. Restrooms are in the building directly across the street from the office.

walk 17
Calvary Cemetery

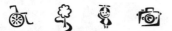

General location: North of Interstate 70 in the northeast part of the city.

Special attractions: Ornate monuments and mausoleums, park setting and lush landscaping, historic gravesites of some of the city's most notable residents.

Difficulty rating: Easy, flat, entirely on paved roadways.

Distance: 2 miles.

Estimated time: 1.5 hours.

Services: Restrooms and water are available at the main entrance. The restrooms are not wheelchair-accessible.

Restrictions: Although this is a private cemetery, visitors are invited to enjoy the beautiful grounds and the rich history captured here. However, please remember that these grounds are a place for serenity and reflection.

For more information: Contact Calvary Cemetery.

Getting started: Take Interstate 70 to the West Florissant Exit 245B. Then go north on Florissant for about half a mile. Turn right onto Calvary Avenue and park near the main office, where a free map of the grounds is available.

Public transportation: Bi-State Transit Bus 95 stops on West Florissant near the cemetery entrance. Contact Bi-State for information on schedules and fares.

Overview: Calvary Cemetery is a tad younger than Bellefontaine, its neighbor to the south; at almost 480 acres, it is also larger. Although established in 1857, it contains the graves of people who died much earlier but were buried first in Catholic cemeteries that were closed when the growing city needed more room downtown. Like Bellefontaine, Calvary is the final resting place for many well-known citizens of St. Louis. The two cemeteries share not only a common street boundary, Calvary Avenue, but also an attractive parklike setting, curving roadways, intricate memorial art, towering monuments, and architecturally noteworthy mausoleums.

The walk

Most of the roadways in Calvary do not have marked street names. Instead, the cemetery uses section numbers to help people locate graves. These section numbers are often painted prominently on the curbing or noted on brass markers placed near the roadways. During this walk, you will often be able to determine your location by noting nearby section markers as they are mentioned in the text.

►This walk starts by the cemetery office on Calvary Avenue, just inside the gates. Walk northeast on Calvary toward the large brown building you see down the road.

Calvary Cemetery

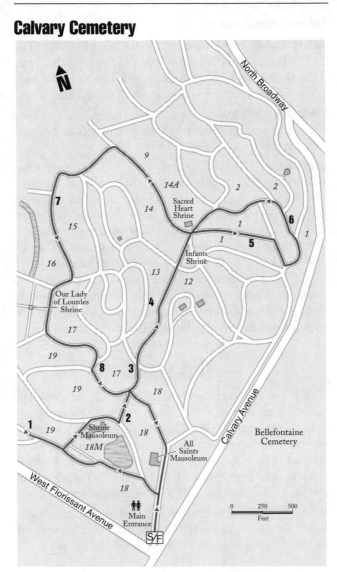

Calvary Cemetery

1	Thomas A. Dooley	5	Dred Scott
2	Vivand Family	6	Antoine Soulard
3	General William T. Sherman	7	Tennessee Williams
4	Tierre Chouteau	8	Kate Chopin

➤Turn left at the first intersection. You will be walking toward the lake and will see Section 18 on the curbs to your left and right.

➤At the Y intersection by the lake, take the left arm of the Y. You will see many unique monument structures not only in this area, but also elsewhere along this walk. Inspect those tombs and gravesites that attract your attention, but be sure to return where you left the road.

➤At the intersection of three roadways, where you see the James Morgan mausoleum on your left, take either of the two paths directly in front of you. They will merge at their other end.

➤Where the two roads converge, continue straight ahead. To your right you will see the metal Way of Galilee Section 19 cemetery marker and rows of uniform monuments in the new priests' lot. This is where priests from the Archdiocese of St. Louis are now buried. The Shrine Mausoleum will also be to your right at the intersection where you go straight ahead.

➤Stop by a large tree with a ground-level monument that depicts the crucified Christ. This is the grave of Dr. Thomas A. Dooley, who wrote several books in the 1950s on his medical assistance to the people of Southeast Asia. They gave many Americans their first look at this part of the world and made Dooley a household name.

➤Retrace your steps back to the intersection by the Shrine Mausoleum.

➤Turn left and walk between the priests' burial lot and the gray granite mausoleum. You might want to visit the mausoleum and view the stained glass windows in its chapel.

➤At the T intersection, turn right. Directly in front of you as you make this right-hand turn will be a large cross with the name McNichols, a carved child on the Kirns marker, and a dramatic angel holding a cross.

➤As you approach the next intersection, note the large markers in front of you. Tall and close together, they look like buildings in a miniature city. The lake will be visible on your right.

➤Walk toward the guardian angel statue on the Viviano family tomb. The Vivianos began as pastatiers at the turn of the century. The monument's four columns represent the four brothers who founded the company.

➤Turn left in front of the Viviano monument. You will see Section 19 on the curb to your left and a step monument with the name Walker.

➤Walk toward the four-way intersection. You can see that the road you are on will curve after you cross the intersection.

➤Angle toward the Siemers family marker, which is an angel standing in front of the cross, and continue on the curving roadway. Look for a flagpole coming up on your left.

➤Walk toward the flagpole and the collection of markers. This is the family burial site of Union General William Tecumseh Sherman.

➤Return to the roadway with Sherman's grave to your left. You are now facing three road choices.

➤Take the middle fork. The curb sign for Section 13 will come up directly in front of you. As you walk along this middle fork, look off to your left for an elevated piece of ground. A marble stairway ascends this small hill and leads to a circular courtyard filled with monuments. In the middle is a cross surrounded by a large pile of rocks.

➤Go up the steps to the small balcony and the family plot of Pierre Chouteau, son of St. Louis founder Pierre de Laclède and Marie Thérèse Chouteau, his wife except by law. In this Catholic region, Madame Chouteau was unable to divorce her estranged husband, Rene Auguste Chouteau. She had four children with Laclède, but by law all had to be recorded as the children of Chouteau.

Pierre and a half-brother, Auguste Chouteau, gained wealth and prestige by trading successfully for furs with the Indians, especially the Osage. The Osage so respected the brothers that they adopted them into their clans. When he was 91, Pierre Chouteau died in the cholera epidemic of 1849. When you are through exploring this gravesite, go down the stairs and return to where you left the road.

➤At the next four-way intersection, continue straight ahead. On your right, in the middle on a triangular-shaped plot, you will see a tiny sculpture. This small marker rests in the Infants Shrine, the tiny burial spot for children.

➤Continue past the Infants Shrine. At the end of the grassy area, bypass the sharply angled right road. You will see curb signs for Section 1 in front of you and to your right.

➤Take the next road to the right. On your left as you make this right-hand turn, you will see a sign for Section 14A. Behind you is a large statue with its back to you. You are walking away from the statue and into a more open area. After you enter this area of the cemetery, you will see a brass marker for Section 1 Lot K on your right. Shortly after you pass the marker, you will see a series a crosses on the right that mark the graves of members of the Sisters Servants of the Holy Spirit of Perpetual Adoration. When you pass these graves, begin to look for a monument that is about three

Dred Scott

Dred Scott's burial stone says he was born about 1799, was freed by his friend Taylor Blow, and died September 17, 1858. Space does not allow the stone to tell the larger story.

Slaves Dred Scott and his wife, Harriet, sued for their freedom in the circuit court of St. Louis. Their lawyer argued that because both had spent long periods of time in the free territories of Illinois and what is now Minnesota, they could no longer be slaves in Missouri. The lower court, which had granted freedom to slaves in similar situations, agreed with them. But by the time the Supreme Court of Missouri heard the owner's appeal in 1852, slavery had become much more controversial, and the state supreme court reversed the decision.

Some suggest that through procedural error and a feigned desire on the part of the owner to hold on to the slaves, the case moved to the U.S. Supreme Court. Those for and against slavery wanted the court to hear the case.

In 1857, the U.S. Supreme Court ruled that blacks, whether enslaved or free, were not citizens. It also ruled that under the Fifth Amendment to the U.S. Constitution, citizens could not be deprived of their property, human or otherwise, simply because they stepped into free territory. The Missouri Compromise was declared unconstitutional, and the Civil War moved closer.

As for the Scotts, they were sold to Taylor Blow, a man Dred had grown up with, for a negligible amount. Blow then set the Scotts free. They returned to the courthouse where eleven years earlier they had first sued for their freedom. This time, however, they came to register themselves as free Negroes. Dred died the next year.

feet tall and on your right. The back of the stone will carry the name of Dred Scott and an inscription: "Subject of the decision of the Supreme Court of the United States in 1857, which denied citizenship to the Negro. Voided the Missouri Compromise that became one of the events that resulted in the Civil War."

➤Continue past Scott's grave.

➤At the T intersection, turn right.

➤Follow the road as it curves to the left, bypassing a road that comes in from the right. When you have completed the curve, you will come to a Y intersection.

➤Take the left arm of the Y. Look to your right in the Y-shaped plot of ground for an obelisk with a cross on its top. Just beyond this obelisk in Section 3 is the monument to Antoine Soulard, a French naval lieutenant and the King's Surveyor for upper Louisiana. Soulard married Julia Cerré, the youngest daughter of Gabriel Cerré, a wealthy merchant and one of the city's founding fathers. Her social standing and inheritance, plus Soulard's position of influence, combined to make the Soulards a powerful St. Louis family.

Note the nearby monument with a fallen cross on it. It is the grave of Charles Gratiot, himself a member of an early and prominent St. Louis family. Take a moment to walk through this area. The graves are old, and many of the stones have been worn away. Just be sure to go back to the roadway that passes directly in front of Soulard's monument.

➤When you have returned to the roadway, continue northward on the path that brought you here.

➤Walk toward the intersection and take its left curve. Section 1 is on the curb markers to your left, and the Witte obelisk is to your left as you approach this left-hand curve.

➤Keep to your left. Section 1 will be on the left curb and Section 2, which has its own brass marker, will be across the street. To your left you should see the gray granite, square tombstone of Maxwell, followed by an obelisk with a funeral drape on top.

➤Continue on this road as it meanders, keeping the Section 1 markers to your left. You should pass a brass marker with Section 1 Lot 643 on your left, and just beyond that will be a red granite truncated cross.

➤At the four-way intersection, bear left. The Section 1 marker on your left will say "Way of Bethany." As you make the left turn, several brass markers will come on your left. One will say Section 1 Lot L, another Section 1 Lot 0. The angled look of these markers suggests that occasionally people may try to remove them. Shortly after you pass the marker for Lot 0, you will come to the intersection of several roads.

➤Stop for a moment to get your bearings. To your left is the curb marker for Section 1. Immediately to your right is the marker for Section 14A.

➤Take the road to your right that goes between Section 14A and Section 14. To your right and in front of you is the statue and shrine to the Sacred Heart.

➤Continue down this road with the Sacred Heart to your right and a sweeping hillside to your left. You will go for a few blocks; take in the sights and enjoy the quiet drama of this area.

➤Turn left where you see a low stone wall with markers. Section 14B will be on the curb in front of the wall. Behind you is Section 9.

➤At the next intersection, Section 15 is in front of you under a tree.

➤Take the road that curves right. Two other roads branch to the left. The Section 15 curb marker will be in front of you as you curve to the right.

➤Follow the road as it bends left.

➤Continue straight ahead, staying to the left. Shortly after you see Section 15A, you will come upon the grave of poet and playwright Tennessee Williams. His plays include *The Glass Menagerie*, and the Pulitzer Prize winning plays *A Streetcar Named Desire* and *Cat on a Hot Tin Roof*. His monument carries the inscription: "The violets in the mountains have broken the rocks." Next to him rests Rose Isabelle Williams, whose inscription reads, "Blow out your candles, Laura."

➤Continue straight ahead. To your left are monuments; to your right is a wooded area that opens up again into an expanse of grass.

➤At the T intersection, with Section 17 directly in front of you, turn right. You will pass the Our Lady of Lourdes Shrine on your right.

➤This road will curve to your left and you will see Section 17A directly in front of you. As the names on the monuments indicate, you are now walking through the Italian section.

➤At the Y intersection the curb and brass markers in front of you say Section 19.

➤Take the left arm of the Y. As you near the next intersection, look to your left for the large Cummings memorial site. You are looking for the gravesite of novelist Kate Chopin, who died in 1904. Her grave is in the grass and to the left of the Cummings memorial. *The Republic*, a St. Louis newspaper, once described Chopin as the "most brilliant, distinguished, and interesting woman who ever graced

of interest

Symbols in the stone

Messages of sorrow, love, and hope often are encoded in monument art. As you roam historic Calvary and Bellefontaine Cemeteries, see if you can decipher the sentiments of the living when they selected the ornamentation for their loved ones' graves. These examples may help.

Angel: rebirth, protection, wisdom, mercy, Divine love
Sleeping angel: innocence
Bell: mourning
Broken sword: life cut short
Celtic cross: faith and eternity
Columns: noble life
Cross: faith, resurrection
Door: entrance to heaven
Female form: sorrow, grief
Flag: military, patriotism
Harp: hope
Heart: love, devotion
Lamb: resurrection
Lily: purity, sometimes chastity
Obelisk: rebirth, connection between heaven and earth
Palm leaves: victory over death, righteousness
Tree stump: shortness of life
Urn: immortality, penitence

St. Louis." Her novel *The Awakening*, with its description of a married woman's love affair, shocked readers in the late 1800s. As you leave Chopin's grave, you might want to explore the large and elaborate Cummings memorial.

➤When you leave the Cummings plot, the Section 19 curb marker and the T. Ward memorial stone should face you.

➤Take the road that goes to the left. On your right as you make the turn, you will see the Hau Schulte obelisk and an enclosed walled area with two carved churches—the Joseph O'Neil memorial site. As you walk a little farther along this left-curving road, you will see the lake and All Saints Mausoleum off to your right.

➤At the intersection, continue straight ahead. You will encounter your first sidewalk since beginning this walk. To the left is the large Slevin obelisk. The monuments in this area are all larger than life.

➤Follow the sidewalk as it passes the All Saints Mausoleum.

➤The cemetery gates are now visible, and you can return to your car. The restrooms can be reached from the outside of the office. The path to the restrooms is wheelchair-accessible, but the facilities are not.

If cemetery art intrigues you, you may enjoy the book *Soul in the Stone: Cemetery Art in America* by writer and photographer John Gary Brown. The book contains many memorials found in these cemeteries.

Our Lady of the Snows Shrine

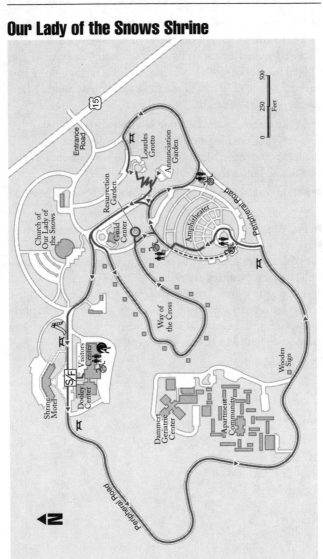

walk 18

Our Lady of the Snows Shrine

General location: Fifteen minutes east of downtown St. Louis in Belleville, Illinois.

Special attractions: One of the country's largest outdoor shrines, beautifully landscaped grounds.

Difficulty rating: On paved, wide roadways but with some hills. The path is wheelchair-accessible, but wheelchair users may need assistance on the long, steady inclines. All buildings and facilities are accessible.

Distance: 2.5 miles.

Estimated time: 1.5 hours.

Services: The Shrine Motel, and restrooms, religious gift shop, and restaurant in the St. Joseph Visitors Center. Tram tours available.

193

Restrictions: Walk during daylight hours.

For more information: Contact the National Shrine of Our Lady of the Snows or the Belleville Tourism Division.

Getting started: Take Interstate 55 east out of downtown St. Louis to I-64. Go east on I-64 and take the I-255 South exit. Follow I-255 to Exit 17A and State Road 15. Follow SR 15 two miles to the shrine. Turn right into the shrine and follow the signs to the visitor center and ample parking.

Public transportation: None.

Overview: Each year almost 1 million people visit this 200-acre shrine, which was founded in 1958 by Father Edwin J. Guild, a member of the Missionary Oblates of Mary Immaculate. On these carefully manicured grounds you will find a 2,400-seat amphitheater, a replica of the Lourdes Grotto, prayer gardens and chapels, the Way of the Cross, and statuary. Most of the shrine's programs are ecumenical in spirit and supported by people of all faiths. Towering trees, colorful seasonal flowers, and a peaceful, gracious atmosphere add to the shrine's ambiance.

During the Christmas season—the day after Thanksgiving through New Year's—the shrine hosts its annual Way of Lights, a nightly, decorative light display that leads car visitors on a "Journey to Bethlehem." Visitors travel past almost a million glittering white lights, illuminated life-size statues and lighted art sculptures on their way to the Nativity, which is tucked into a natural cave. Weather permitting, visitors can take a horse-drawn carriage or a tram through the light display.

The walk

➤You will start at the St. Joseph's Visitors Center. Leave the center and walk toward the road.

➤Turn left onto the roadway. For about a mile, this wide peripheral road will be your walking path. Traffic is light through the shrine, but watch for cars. The sweet gum trees that line the first part of the path will give way to towering trees, evergreens, seasonal flowering shrubs and trees, and dense vegetation—all set back from the road. You will find no shade on a sunny day. Follow the gentle, but continuous incline through this park setting. Soon you will see the satellite dishes of the Apartment Community.

➤Continue on the peripheral road as it skirts the Apartment Community and the Dammert Geriatric Center.

➤At the stop-sign intersection, continue straight ahead. On your left you will pass a large wooden sign that guides oncoming cars toward the apartments and geriatric center.

➤You will walk through an open area with a large expanse of green lawn and head downhill toward the arches of the amphitheater and outdoor altar.

➤Turn left into the driveway of the amphitheater and walk between two stone angels. In June, peonies will be in bloom here.

➤Enter the building and follow the hall to your right as it winds past the Christ the King Chapel, lit candles, and mosaics. You will pass a unisex restroom at the end of the votive candles.

Note: If you are pushing a wheelchair, a few steps will prevent you from using this route to enter the arena area. Instead, follow the roadway on the building's west side, which will give you access to the amphitheater and altar area.

➤After you pass the votive wall, walk up a few steps and into the arena.

➤Turn left and walk between the seats and the stage.

➤Follow the wide aisle as it angles to your right and up to the amphitheater's upper level. You are heading up a short but steep hill toward the drinking fountain and restroom, which will be on your left. A curb in front of the restroom area may make this restroom difficult for wheelchair users.

➤Continue on the path as it leads away from the amphitheater. The sign indicates that the visitor tour is to your left and the Annunciation Garden is to the right.

➤Follow the right curve and the path to the Annunciation Garden. From here you get a nice view of the amphitheater.

➤Follow the path into the Annunciation Garden, which is vibrant with iris and azalea in the spring and roses in the summer. Hosta and other greenery decorate the borders. Explore the Father's Memorial Wall, which is to your left, and the Mother's Prayer Wall, which is ahead and to your right. Both of these areas include personal plaques and remembrances.

The larger-than-life statues representing the Annunciation are directly ahead and just beyond the vibrant blue reflection pool. The four bells resting above the water ring out on the hour and dramatically break the stillness.

➤Take the path back to where you entered the garden and turn left onto the roadway.

➤Follow the road as it curves to your left.

➤Turn into Lourdes Grotto, a smaller replica of the grotto in France. You will find picnic tables, many benches, and racks of candles. To your right and toward the altar area is a drinking fountain and a trail that goes to the Father's Memorial Wall.

➤Take that zigzag path. This paved forest trail is especially lovely in the fall. Honeysuckle and wild daisies decorate the pathway in the spring. Poison oak and ivy are troublesome

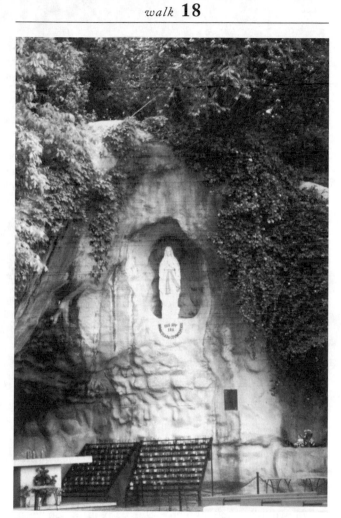

The Lourdes Grotto at Our Lady of the Snows Shrine provides a place for reflection.

year-round, so stay on the trail. At the top of the switchback you will find a bench, a good spot to stop and catch your breath.

➤At the top, turn right and head to the road. The Annunciation Garden is directly behind you.

➤Turn right onto the road and walk toward the Edwin J. Guild Center.

➤At the Guild Center, follow the road as it curves to your left and heads toward the Way of the Cross, which is set in a grove of evergreens. Station 1 will come up on your right. The statues at each of the fourteen stations capture a particular moment during the Passion.

➤After you pass Station 14, cross the road and enter Resurrection Garden. Here you will find a cave with the inscription: "He is not here, for He is risen." The tomb's interior—a cut geode—sparkles and houses a perpetual flame that appears and disappears, depending on where you stand.

➤Turn left when you leave the garden.

➤Turn left again, and yet again as you follow the road that heads toward the Guild Center and away from the amphitheater. You may want to stop in the center and see "The Journey," a twenty-minute sound-and-light show that the shrine describes as "a pilgrimage through creation, the fall, and humanity's search for meaning and redemption."

➤When you pass or leave the Guild Center, take the second road curving to your left. The first road goes to the Way of the Cross.

➤You will pass the Church of Our Lady of the Snows on your right and on your left, the Agony Garden, located in a dense grove of trees.

➤Follow the road back to the visitor center and your car.

walk 19
St. Charles

General location: Thirty minutes west of downtown St. Louis off Interstate 70.

Special attractions: Nine-block historic district, riverboat entertainment, nineteenth-century architecture, quaint shops, antique stores, museums, Shrine of St. Rose Philippine Duchesne.

Difficulty rating: Easy, all on concrete and brick sidewalks, but with some uneven surfaces and hills.

Distance: 2.3 miles.

Estimated time: 1.5 hours.

Services: Restrooms along route in restaurants and museums; information, water, and restrooms in St. Charles Tourism Center.

Restrictions: Dogs must be leashed and droppings picked up.

St. Charles

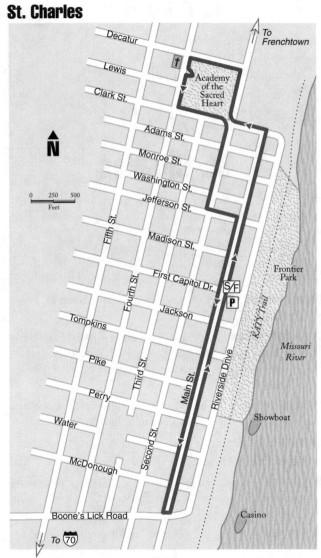

For more information: Contact the St. Charles Convention and Visitors Bureau, which is located in the St. Charles Tourism Center.

Getting started: From Interstate 70, take the Fifth Street exit and follow Fifth north to First Capitol Drive. Turn right and drive toward the river. After you cross South Main Street, look for the parking lot entrance coming up on your right. Parking is free.

Public transportation: None.

Overview: This historic town was founded in the late 1760s by Louis Blanchette and a group of Creole hunters. Its first name—Les Petites Côtes—came from the small hills that afforded the area some protection along the Missouri River. Rich in game, with fertile land, the area prospered.

During Spanish rule, the village was known as San Carlos de Misuri. With the Louisiana Purchase in 1804, the village's Spanish name was simply translated to St. Charles. That year Meriwether Lewis and William Clark camped here for five days before heading westward to explore the Louisiana Purchase.

In 1821, when Missouri was admitted to the Union, St. Charles became the state's first capital. It held that position until 1826, when the state government moved to Jefferson City.

Today this city of about 54,600 people welcomes almost a million visitors a year. People come to walk the historic district with its brick streets, gaslights, and nineteenth-century buildings. Strollers find more than one hundred specialty and antique stores and dozens of interesting restaurants, many with patio dining. At the river they can enjoy gaming or Broadway shows on a riverboat.

The town's annual festivals are also popular. The Lewis and Clark Rendezvous, which reenacts the explorers' encampment, is held the third weekend in May. Fife and drum corps, black-powder shoots, and crafts and costumes take St. Charles back to 1804. The Festival of the Little Hills is held in mid-August and celebrated with crafts and food. Oktoberfest, held the first weekend in October, honors the town's German heritage with music, food, and art.

The walk

➤From the parking lot at the corner of Riverside and First Capitol Drives, cross First Capitol and enter the back door of the St. Charles Tourism Center. Be sure to stop by the front desk and request information about the South Main Street Walking Tour. With its delightful architectural drawings and wealth of historic information on the buildings along South Main, the packet is well worth a donation.

➤Turn right when you leave the center's front door. As you pass the archway over the path leading to the river, try to imagine this town when river steamers were commercial lifelines. Crews would unload cargo into carriages that would then haul goods to Main Street's waiting merchants. The first steamboat came by in 1818, the last in 1992!

The three buildings under one roof at #208-216 housed the state's first capitol. This historic site is open daily, so pop in and look around. You will find journal entries from Meriwether Lewis. On May 20, 1804, he wrote, "St. Charles is bisected by one principle street, about a mile in length running nearly parallel to the river....The village contains a chapel, 100 dwelling houses and about 450 inhabitants who are principally descendants of Canadian French."

➤Walk down Main to Clark Street. Main ends here and the American Car and Foundry Company will be on the northwest corner.

➤Cross Clark and turn left.

➤At the four-way stop at Second Street and Clark, cross Second. You are standing at the southeast corner of the Shrine of St. Rose Philippine Duchesne and the Academy of the Sacred Heart. The shrine's entrance is off of Fourth Street, and this walk will take you there.

➤Go to your right and walk one block north along Second and the shrine grounds.

of interest

St. Philippine Duchesne

Philippine Duchesne, a French sister and pioneer saint in the Society of the Sacred Heart, felt driven to serve as a missionary in the New World. In 1818, she and a small group of sisters opened the Academy of the Sacred Heart, the first free school established west of the Mississippi River. The original log cabin is gone, but primitive remains from those early school days are on exhibit in the museum. Today the school educates about seven hundred elementary school children.

On July 3, 1988, Mother Duchesne was canonized in the Roman Catholic Church and became the fourth U.S. saint. The shrine, which includes her stone coffin, attracts pilgrims from around the world. The Missouri granite in the sanctuary is symbolic of the rugged pioneer life she endured.

The wall hanging seen in the choir loft is a reproduction of the stained glass window in a church in Mound City, Kansas, where she worked among the Potawatomi Indians. This banner hung outside Rome's St. Peter's Basilica the morning of her canonization.

➤At Decatur Street, turn left. The path has a slight incline. Note the sign with an arrow that points down Second in the direction of Frenchtown. This neighborhood is known for its antique stores and also for fifty-eight preserved buildings of French Colonial and German architecture. After your walk, you may want to explore this section of St. Charles.

➤At Fourth Street and Decatur, turn left. Across the street is the St. Charles Boromeo Church, with its high spires and stained glass. The town was named for this saint. The homes in this neighborhood are old and charming. Note the pale yellow house across the street. With its banisters and large open porch, it suggests something French.

➤Continue down Fourth. The shrine entrance will come up on your left in the middle of the block.

➤Follow the sign that points toward the shrine, which is tucked in and behind the buildings facing Fourth. The shrine is open for daily visitation. Contact the shrine office for information about guided tours and services.

➤When you leave the shrine, turn left on Fourth.

➤Walk one block to Clark and turn left. Note the old homes in this neighborhood.

➤At Second and Clark, turn right, cross Clark, and continue on Second. The new building on your right is the St. Charles County Justice Center and across the street is the county's Courts Administration Building.

➤Continue down Second four blocks to Jefferson Street. At the corner of Jefferson and Second you have quite a view. Immediately to your right is the domed St. Charles County Courthouse, built in 1904. In the distance to your left is the Missouri River and the many old buildings that still give this city its frontier feel.

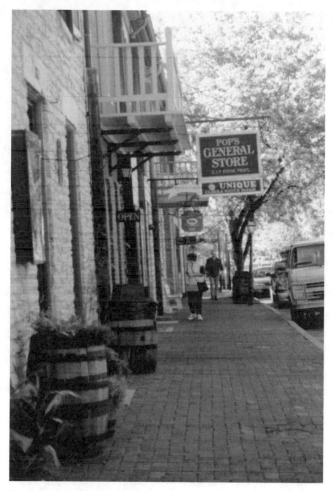

Brick sidewalks, gaslights, and quaint shops add to the charm of St. Charles.

The sign in front of the county building notes that you are standing on a major crossroads. Many feet have trod this ground: Indians, then hunters and trappers, and even Daniel Boone, who discovered a salt springs along this part of the trail. The early highway became known as Boone's Lick Road. Later the Santa Fe Trail, the Salt Lake Trail, and the great Oregon Trail passed through here.

►At the corner of Second and Jefferson, turn left and go toward the river to Main Street. On your right, notice the red-brick building with the ornamental grillwork and birds, and stained glass windows.

►At Main and Jefferson, turn right. The brick building on the corner, #101, was built in 1832 and houses the Archives of the St. Charles County Historical Society.

►You will walk along this side of Main for nine blocks. Along the way you will see wooden rain spouts, whiskey barrels with a second life as trash cans, and maybe even horse-drawn carriages, which do not seem a bit out of place. In the early days, this street was the village's commercial and residential district, for merchants sold goods and services from their homes.

At #337, note the carved columns and lintels. Stonecutter Joseph May built this house around 1870. The walking tour guide notes that the first floor slopes toward the street, so May would have an easier time rolling his finished works out the door.

In the 1800s, the entire 500 block of this side of Main was known as Tavern Square and was the center of town until the 1860s. Number 515, built in the 1820s, was a tavern known as the St. Charles Hotel.

All the buildings on either side of the 700 block are original and date to the 1800s. The Federal-style house at #701-703 was built around the 1820s. The land may have been

of interest

Explore the KATY Trail

In 1986, the Missouri-Kansas-Texas (MKT) Railroad, known as the KATY, abandoned more than 200 miles of rail line in central Missouri. With the help of the Natural Trails Systems Act and private funds, the Missouri Department of Natural Resources was able to convert the railroad bed into a relatively flat Rails-to-Trails path for walkers and bikers of all ages and abilities.

The KATY Trail, one of the longest continuous Rails-to-Trails conversions in the country, starts in St. Charles and continues west to Sedalia. More than 160 miles of the trail follows the Missouri River, giving walkers and bicyclists spectacular views of the river and the one-hundred-foot bordering bluffs.

Located along the Missouri River flyway, the trail attracts migrating birds and waterfowl. Rock formations, wild flowers, bottomland and upland forests, wetlands, farmland, and wineries bring year-round beauty and interest. The trail has also brought a rebirth to the tiny towns that once flourished with the railroads and then declined with their departure.

In St. Charles, the trail begins in Frontier Park, between Riverside Drive and the Missouri River—just feet from the Tourism Center. The trail is just behind the solitary caboose.

The KATY may go for miles, but most walkers cover only a few miles before retracing their route back to their cars. Bikers, however, can go the distance; many towns cater to these long-distance travelers. If you would like more information on the services—bed and breakfasts, restaurants, bike rentals, and transportation shuttles—located along the KATY, contact the Missouri Department of Natural Resources or the KATY Trail Merchants Group.

owned by the town's founder, Louis Blanchette. Number 709 was once a blacksmith shop, and the large, curved window was the shop entrance for carriages and wagons.

➤Turn left at Boone's Lick Road, cross Main, and walk along Main's east side. Boone's Lick Road started at this intersection, and thousands left from this spot for points as far west as California.

The Lewis and Clark 1804 rendezvous site is at this end of Main; and depending on when you walk, you might catch the sound of pipe and drum music. You should also catch great aromas coming from restaurant kitchens.

➤You will follow this side of Main to First Capitol Drive.

Stop at the corner of Main and Perry. A river ferry once operated at the foot of Perry, and many travelers coming into town along Perry stayed at a hotel located at 700 Main. The Lewis and Clark Center, a museum tracing the explorers' trip, is just down Perry at 701 Riverside.

➤Turn right when you reach First Capitol Drive and return to the parking lot and your car.

walk 20
Laumeier Sculpture Park

General location: Twelve miles southwest of downtown St. Louis.

Special attractions: Modern art displayed in a park setting on the grounds of an old estate.

Difficulty rating: Easy, primarily flat and on paved surfaces with some hard-packed dirt and a short incline. Those pushing strollers or using wheelchairs have a flat, all-paved, out-and-back option. The out-and-back trail has no shade.

Distance: 0.75 mile for the closed-loop trail that includes a short stretch of dirt and grass in the woods; 1 mile for the all-paved, out-and-back walk.

Estimated time: 1 hour.

Services: Restrooms in the museum and along paved trail, outdoor patio and benches for picnicking. During museum

Laumeier Sculpture Park

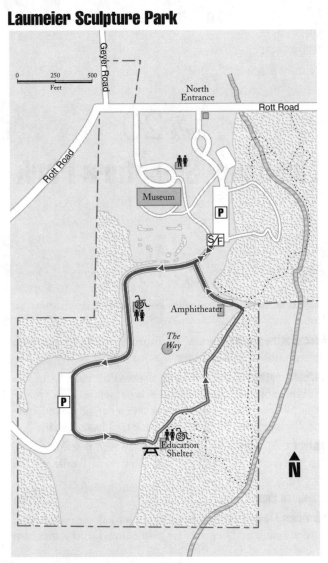

hours, visitors may borrow an audio cassette guide that describes the sculptures.

Restrictions: No climbing on sculptures.

For more information: Contact the Laumeier Sculpture Park.

Getting started: Take Interstate 44 east or west to the Lindbergh Boulevard exit. Go half a mile south on Lindbergh to Rott Road. Turn right on Rott and go half a mile to the park entrance, which will be on your left. Follow the road into the parking lot; parking is easier to find in the morning. If you accidentally pass the first entrance, you will find a second entrance on your left. However, this entrance is only open during museum hours. You cannot reach the parking lot from the museum entrance, but you can park in the driveway and walk down to the parking lot where this walk starts.

Public transportation: Bi-State Transit Bus 11 goes along Rott Road by the park. Bus 11 starts at the downtown bus terminal at Broadway and Locust; Rott Road is at the route's far western end. Call Bi-State to confirm the schedule.

Overview: Founded in 1976, Laumeier Sculpture Park was among the first contemporary sculpture parks in the United States. Created from the estate of millionaires Henry and Matilda Laumeier, it exhibits and preserves large-scale outdoor sculpture in a natural setting. Some consider Laumeier the world's premier park for site sculpture.

In this ninety-six-acre St. Louis County park, you will find sculptures along hiking trails in peaceful woodlands, by paved walking paths, and in expansive, sun-drenched meadows. Smaller works in other media—such as ceramics, painting and photography—also are on display in the Laumeier museum galleries.

With a mix of sculptures that are either permanently installed or on loan, seasonal fairs and festivals that showcase national artists, and special exhibits, Laumeier's ensures a variety of art throughout the year. Its Contemporary Art and Craft Fair in mid-May, summer concerts, and the children's art festivals are popular events. The park is free, though some special events may charge admission.

The walk

➤Start this walk at the south end of the parking lot, which is located between the woods and the large stone house that serves as the park's office and museum. This was the Laumeiers' home. If you are starting your walk when the museum is open, you may want to get the self-guided tour map, which will give you the names of the sculptures you will be seeing from a distance.

At this end of the parking lot, near the start of the paved trail, you will find maquettes, or small models, for three much larger sculptures. A sculptor creates a maquette (pronounced ma-KET) as a way to examine a work's overall design from many perspectives before beginning the actual construction. The three models are for *Triangular Bridge Over Water* by Dan Graham; *Cromlech Glen*, a massive earth work by Beverly Pepper; and *Untitled* by Ursula Von Rydingsvard, an orderly arrangement of wooden rectangles. You can find the full-sized sculptures in the woods to your left.

Maquettes give visitors a more intimate and up-close look at a work. They also offer those with sight impairments the opportunity to explore the sculptures with their hands and to literally grasp the overall work. The descriptions for these maquettes, and others in the park, are written in braille as well as standard text.

➤Head off to your right on the walking path. On your left

you will see *Ada's Will* by Jene Highstein. The maquette for this sculpture is on your right.

➤The first paved trail coming up on your left goes to the amphitheater. If you are doing the loop walk, you will come back on this path and will get a closer look at the sculptures along that route.

On your right is a collection of several works, both permanent and on loan. You may want to explore these now. You can also walk among these sculptures or view many of them from the museum's patio at the end of this walk.

➤Continue on the trail. The tall work of several figures in a row is *Solstice* by William King. On your left is *Two Standing Poets* by Ernest Trova. It was Trova's search for a permanent home for his sculpture collection that enabled these grounds to make the transition from a county park to an outdoor sculpture museum. Laumeier's permanent collection includes seventeen Trova works.

To your left is an immense arrangement of red drums that from a distance resemble some ancient ruin. This is *The Way* by Alexander Liberman, the park's signature piece. You may want to walk out to it, run your hands along its smooth sides, and feel small in its presence.

➤Accessible restrooms are coming up on your left. *The Way* maquette will be on your left after the restrooms.

➤Follow the trail into the parking lot and pick it up again at the other end. Arranged around the lot are *Rolling Explosion*, with its big wheels and tracks, by Dennis Oppenheim; *Untitled*, a ground-hugging work by Robert Morris; and *Untitled*, an arrangement of squares by Donald Judd.

➤At the south end of the parking lot, walk through the three wooden posts and follow the path toward the woods.

To your right in the open area are several works, some of which are on loan.

➤You will come to the Education Shelter, which is used for art camp. Here you will find water, accessible restrooms, and picnic tables.

➤Continue on the asphalt trail past the education shelter. You are now in the woods. The asphalt trail will end where you see a bench on your left. If you are pushing a stroller or using a wheelchair, you may want to retrace your path back to the start point. However, the next half-mile stretch of dirt, followed by some grass, is fairly compact. Except for one incline, this wide dirt and gravel trail is also fairly level and manageable. However, if it has rained recently, the trail may be muddy and not worth the effort.

➤The trail marker points ahead to the amphitheater, which is where you are going.

➤Do not take any trails coming up on your right.

➤Go left at the first intersection where you can turn left. You will encounter a steep, but short hill. You are now on a grassy area behind the amphitheater.

➤Get on the paved trail that is on your right as you face the back of the stage.

➤Follow this paved path.

➤When the path ends, turn right and return to your car.

If you want to explore the museum and small gift shop, follow the sidewalk heading off to your left. An accessible path leads to the back patio, and from there you can follow the accessible route into the building. You may want to linger on the patio and savor the view or find a nearby bench and enjoy a picnic, if you have brought one. You may purchase beverages in the museum.

of interest

Art in the woods

The paved paths in Laumeier Sculpture Park offer a wonderful opportunity to experience art in a natural setting and to enjoy a delightful place in which to stroll. The park's many wooded walking paths, however, offer yet another experience—the chance to discover art under the canopy of an urban forest. Laumeier's well-deserved reputation as a premier sculpture park comes, in part, from its effort to find works that blend with the natural setting, including a woods.

The dirt trails heading off from the east parking lot meander among the trees and take you to monumental surprises. Here sculptures pop out from around a bend in the trail, straddle a creek bed, stretch out in a clearing, or become part of a grand, but long-abandoned swimming pool. They stand silently like Mayan temples or solidly as a mass of earth.

These woods are lovely, peaceful, and perfect for a quiet walk alone or with friends and family. Children will enjoy the adventure of finding not only the sculptures, but also a stone grotto tucked away under the trees or a burbling creek.

In the spring, the leggy dogwoods with their branches stretched upward burst into bloom; the dappled sunlight dances off their white blossoms. Redbuds and honeysuckle toss in a bit more color. In the summer, the woods offers protection from the sun. Fall and winter bring yet another mix of colors, sounds, and smells.

The trails are well-marked; you should have no trouble finding your way back to the sunlit part of the park. Watch your footing, especially near the old pool, or where the trail is supported by erosion timbers, or when rains have made some spots muddy and slick. Poison ivy lurks, so keep children and pets on the trail.

Appendix A: Other Sights

You may enjoy several other attractions either in or near St. Louis. Some may not involve much walking, but they have been enjoyed by countless tourists and local residents.

In St. Louis

City Museum

701 N. 15th Street

A 70-million-year-old duck-billed dinosaur, caves to explore, a 35,000-gallon aquarium, electric-powered train, and a learning room for preschoolers are just a few of the many unusual items visitors will find in this new downtown museum.

Scott Joplin State Historic Site

2658 Delmar Boulevard

Built shortly after the Civil War, this four-family house was the home of ragtime composer Scott Joplin between 1900 and 1903. It was here that he composed "The Entertainer," made popular by the movie *The Sting*. Visitors will find the restored Joplin flat, African-American history gallery, and visitor center. Call the site for more information.

Grant's Farm

10501 Gravois Road

August A. Busch, Jr. developed this land—once farmed by Ulysses S. Grant—into a country estate. Here the famous Clydesdale horses are bred and trained; more than 1,000 animals from six continents roam free in natural settings.

A tram takes visitors through the grounds, past the wildlife and Grant's cabin, and to the Bauernhof Courtyard where guests receive complementary samples of Anheuser-Busch products or can purchase food and soft drinks.

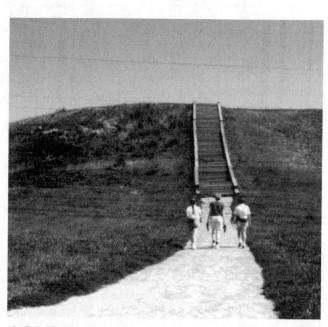

At Cahokia Mounds, many walkers take the stairway to the top of Monks Mound for a view of St. Louis.

You can feed and pet several of the animals, visit the stables, view a carriage collection, or browse in the General Store. The excursion is free, but you must call for reservations.

In the area

Cahokia Mounds

Collinsville, Illinois

A well-kept secret, Cahokia offers a glimpse into the most sophisticated prehistoric Indian civilization found north of Mexico. Inhabited between A.D. 700 and 1400, Cahokia housed about 20,000 people at its peak.

A six-mile self-guided trail winds through the site and takes you to Monk's Mound, the largest prehistoric earthen construction in the New World. Cahokia is such a significant example of human history and culture that the United Nations has declared it a World Heritage Site, a designation shared by such places as China's Great Wall.

A hands-on, child friendly Interpretive Center is filled with artifacts, drawings, and a life-size, walk-through re-creation of a Cahokian neighborhood. Be sure to view "City of the Sun," a fifteen-minute orientation video.

Jefferson Barracks

533 Grant Road

Named for Thomas Jefferson, this military post was established in July 1826, within days of Jefferson's death. Once the nation's largest and most western military post, the barracks protected the wilderness borders and kept peace with the Indians. Its notable soldiers include Jefferson Davis, Robert E. Lee, Ulysses S. Grant, Zachary Taylor, and William T. Sherman.

St. Louis County acquired the post when it was deactivated in 1946. Through the years, the county has restored some of the original buildings—powder magazine museum, laborer's house and stable, and an old ordnance room.

Visitors can walk the self-guided historic tour or almost four miles of paved trails in the adjacent Jefferson Barracks County Park. Jefferson Barracks offers a great outing for kids, many picnic sites, and wonderful bluff views of the Mississippi River. Nearby is historic Jefferson Barracks National Cemetery, the second largest national cemetery.

Appendix B: Contact Information

Throughout this book we have advised you to contact such entities as local attractions, museums, and shops to confirm opening times, locations, and entrance fees. The list below gives you the phone numbers and addresses of all the places we mentioned.

St. Louis

St. Louis Convention and Visitors Commission
One Metropolitan Square, Suite 1100
St. Louis, MO 63102
314-421-1023
800-326-7962
800-916-0040 to request the St. Louis Visitors Guide
www.st-louis-cvc.com

St. Louis Visitors Center
7th Street and Washington Avenue
St. Louis, MO 63101
800-916-0092
> Open Monday through Friday, 9 a.m. to 5 p.m.; Saturday and Sunday, 10 a.m. to 2 p.m.

Activities, Attractions, and Museums

Anheuser-Busch Brewery
13th and Lynch Streets
St. Louis, MO 63118
314-577-2626
> Free tours on a first-come, first-served basis. Open September through May, 9 a.m. to 4 p.m., with tours leaving every 30 minutes. Open June through August, 9 a.m. to 5 p.m., with tours leaving every 10 minutes. Closed Sundays and some holidays.

Bowling Hall of Fame and Museum
11 Stadium Plaza
St. Louis, MO 63102
314-231-6340

Open in the summer from Monday through Saturday, 9 a.m. to 7 p.m.; Sunday, noon to 7 p.m. Closes earlier in winter. Closed Thanksgiving; December 24, 25, and 31; and January 1.

Busch Memorial Stadium and St. Louis Cardinals Hall of Fame
100 Stadium Plaza
St. Louis, MO 63102
314-421-FAME
314-421-3060, ticket information

Stadium tours available. Call for times. Sports Hall of Fame open daily from 10 a.m. to 5 p.m.

Campbell House
1508 Locust Street
St. Louis, MO 63103
314-421-0325

Open Tuesday through Saturday, from 10 a.m. to 4 p.m.; Sunday noon to 5 p.m. Closed January, February, and holidays. Fee for admission.

Chatillon-DeMenil Mansion
3352 DeMenil Place
St. Louis, MO 63118
314-771-5828

Tours are Tuesday through Saturday from 10 a.m. to 4 p.m., with the last tour starting at 3:15 p.m. Lunch is served Tuesday through Saturday.

City Museum

701 North 15th Street
St. Louis, MO 63101
314-241-2489

Open Wednesday through Friday, 9 a.m. to 5 p.m.; Saturday and Sunday, 10 a.m. to 5 p.m. Closed Monday and Tuesday.

Dental Health Theater

727 North First Street
St. Louis, MO 63102
314-241-7391

Open Monday through Friday, 9 a.m. to 4 p.m. Call for show times.

Gateway Riverboat Cruises

Mississippi River below Gateway Arch
314-621-4040
800-878-7411

Cruises daily, April through December.

Grant's Farm

10501 Gravois Road
St. Louis, MO 63123
314-843-1700

Open from April through mid-October. Admission and parking are free, but you must make a reservation.

Jefferson National Expansion Memorial

11 North Fourth Street
St. Louis, MO 63102
314-982-1410

http://www.nps.gov/jeff/arch-home for information on the Gateway Arch, Old Courthouse, or Museum of Westward Expansion.

Arch Tram

Runs daily, except Thanksgiving, Christmas, and New Year's Day. From the Saturday before Memorial Day to Labor Day, trips begin each day at 8:30 a.m. and end with the last trip of the day at 9:10 p.m. On all other days, the first trip is at 9:30 a.m. and the last trip is at 5:10 p.m.

George B. Hartzog Visitor Center in the Gateway Arch

Summer hours 8 a.m. to 10 p.m.; winter hours 9 a.m. to 6 p.m.

Old Courthouse

Open daily from 8 a.m. to 4:30 p.m. To arrange guided tours of the courthouse or dome, call 314-425-6017.

Missouri Botanical Garden

4344 Shaw
St. Louis, MO 63110
314-577-5100, information
314-577-9430, TDD

Open daily from 9 a.m. to 5 p.m., except Christmas. Open from 9 a.m. to 8 p.m., Memorial Day through Labor Day. Grounds open at 7 a.m. Wednesday and Saturday. Fee for admission.

Tower Grove House

Tours daily from 10 a.m. to 4:30 p.m. Closed Thanksgiving, Christmas, and all of January. Fee for admission.

National Video Game and Coin-Op Museum

801 North Second Street
St. Louis, MO 63102
314-621-2900

Open Monday through Saturday, 10 a.m. to 10 p.m.; Sunday, noon to 6 p.m.

Scott Joplin State Historic Site
2658 Delmar Boulevard
St. Louis, MO 63103
314-533-1003
Open April 1 through October 1, Monday through Saturday, 10 a.m. to 5 p.m.; Sunday, noon to 6 p.m. Open the rest of the year, Monday through Saturday, 10 a.m. to 4 p.m.; Sunday, noon to 5 p.m. Closed New Year's Day, Easter, Thanksgiving, and Christmas.

Union Station
Between 18th and 20th Streets Market Street
St. Louis, MO 63103
314-421-6655
Open Monday through Thursday, 10 a.m. to 9 p.m.; Friday and Saturday, 10 a.m. to 10 p.m. (except January through March, when closing time is 9 p.m.); Sunday, 11 a.m. to 7 p.m. (except January through March, when closing time is 6 p.m.). Restaurants may open earlier and close later.

Cemeteries

Bellefontaine Cemetery
4947 West Florissant Avenue
St. Louis, MO 63115
314-381-0750
The cemetery office is open Monday through Friday from 8 a.m. to 4:30 p.m.

Calvary Cemetery
5239 West Florissant Avenue
St. Louis, MO 63115
314-381-1313
The cemetery office is open from 8:30 a.m. to 4:30 p.m. Office is closed Sundays, holidays, and church holy days.

Churches

Cathedral Basilica of Saint Louis
4431 Lindell Boulevard
St. Louis, MO 63108
314-533-2824

> Open to visitors 7 a.m. to dusk, Labor Day to Memorial
> Day; and 7 a.m. to 8 p.m., Memorial Day to Labor Day.
> Tours offered daily at 1 p.m. Mosaics Museum open daily,
> 9 a.m. to 4 p.m.; gift shop open daily, 10 a.m. to 4 p.m.

St. Ambrose Catholic Church
5130 Wilson Avenue
St. Louis, MO 63110
314-771-1228

Sts. Peter and Paul Catholic Church
1919 South Seventh Street
St. Louis, MO 63104
314-231-9923

Trinity Lutheran Church
812 Soulard
St. Louis, MO 63104
314-231-4092

City Parks

Forest Park

314-535-0100

> Open daily, 6 a.m. to 10 p.m. Contact the park for infor-
> mation on golf courses, fishing, tennis courts, and the
> Steinburg Memorial Skating Rink.

Forest Park Boathouse
Government Drive in Forest Park
St. Louis, MO 63110
314-367-3423

Jewel Box
Wells and McKinley Drives in Forest Park
St. Louis, MO 63110
314-531-0080
> Open daily, 9 a.m. to 5 p.m. Free admission Monday and Tuesday from 9 a.m. to noon.

Missouri History Museum
Lindell and DeBaliviere in Forest Park
P.O. Box 11940
St. Louis, MO 63112
314-746-4599
> Open Tuesday, 9:30 a.m. to 8:30 p.m.; Wednesday through Sunday, 9:30 a.m. to 5 p.m. Free admission.

Muny Theater
Forest Park
St. Louis, MO 63112
314-361-1900
> Performances June through August, starting at 8:15 p.m.

St. Louis Art Museum
1 Fine Arts Drive in Forest Park
St. Louis, MO 63110
314-721-0072
> Open Wednesday through Sunday, 10 a.m. to 5 p.m.; Tuesday 1:30 p.m. to 8:30 p.m; tours conducted Wednesday through Sunday at 1:30 p.m. Closed Mondays. Closed Thanksgiving, Christmas, and New Year's Day. Free, but admission charged for special exhibits.

St. Louis Science Center
5050 Oakland Avenue
St. Louis, MO 63110
314-289-4444
800-456-SLSC

Open Monday through Thursday, 9 a.m. to 5 p.m.; Friday,
9 a.m. to 9 p.m.; Saturday, 10 a.m. to 9 p.m; and Sunday,
11 a.m. to 6 p.m. Extended summer hours. Free exhibit
gallery.

St. Louis Zoological Park
1 Government Drive, in Forest Park
St. Louis, MO 63110
314-781-0900
314-768-5421, TDD

Free admission. Open year-round, 9 a.m. to 5 p.m. daily.
Closed Christmas and New Year's Day. From Memorial
Day to Labor Day, open on Tuesdays until 8 p.m.

Tower Grove Park
4255 Arsenal Street
St. Louis, MO 63116
314-771-2679

Park office open Monday through Friday, 8:30 a.m. to 5
p.m.

County Parks

Jefferson Barracks Historic Site
533 Grant Road
St. Louis, MO 63125
314-544-5714

National cemetery is open daily, dawn to dusk. Historic
barracks open Tuesday through Friday, 10 a.m. to 4:30
p.m.; weekends, noon to 4:30 p.m.

Laumeier Sculpture Park
12580 Rott Road
St. Louis, MO 63127
314-821-1209

Open year-round from 7 a.m. to 30 minutes past sunset.
Museum open 10 a.m. to 5 p.m., Tuesday through Saturday;

noon to 5 p.m. on Sunday. Free sculpture tours at 2 p.m. on Sundays, May to October.

Lodging

Lafayette House Bed and Breakfast
2156 Lafayette Avenue
St. Louis, MO 63104
314-772-4429

Schools

Washington University
One Brookings Drive
St. Louis, MO 63130
314-935-5998 (information desk)

Shopping

St. Louis Centre
Washington and 6th Streets
St. Louis, MO 63101
314-231-5913
  Open Monday through Saturday, 10 a.m. to 6 p.m.; Sunday, noon to 5 p.m.

Soulard Farmers Market
730 Carroll
St. Louis, MO 63104
314-622-4180
  Open Wednesday through Saturday.

Transportation

Bi-State Transit
  Customer-service operators available to assist travelers Monday through Friday, 6 a.m. to 8 p.m., and Saturday and Sunday, 8 a.m. to 5 p.m. Out-of-town callers, call

314-231-2345 or 982-1555 for TDD. Callers near St. Louis, but in Illinois, call 271-2345 or 875-1200 for TDD.

MetroLink
Runs from about 5:30 a.m. to midnight, Monday through Saturday, and from 6 a.m. to 11 p.m. on Sunday.

Forest Park Shuttle Bug
Runs from about 6:45 a.m. to 6 p.m. weekdays and from 10 a.m. to 6 p.m. weekends.

Clayton-Galleria Shuttle Bee
Runs from about 5:15 a.m. to midnight weekdays, from about 7 a.m. to 10:30 p.m. on Saturday, and from about 9 a.m. to 7 p.m. Sunday.

Metro Ride Store
St. Louis Centre, street level
7th and Washington Streets
Open Monday through Saturday, 10 a.m. to 6 p.m. Free flyers available outlining every city route, complete with times and stops, plus help from the store's friendly staff. Purchase MetroLink tickets here.

Area Attractions

Belleville, Illinois

Belleville Tourism Division
216 East "A" Street
Belleville, IL 62220
800-677-WALK

National Shrine of Our Lady of the Snows
442 South DeMazenod Drive
Belleville, IL 62223-1094
618-397-6700 or 314-241-3400
www.apci.net/~oblates

Open year-round, 8 a.m. to 10 p.m. Free admission. Visitor center and restaurant closed Christmas Day.

Collinsville, Illinois

Cahokia Mounds Historic Site
Box 681
Collinsville, IL 62234
618-346-5160
Open 9 a.m. to 5 p.m. daily. Closed some holidays.

Collinsville Convention and Visitors Bureau
1 Gateway Drive
Collinsville, IL 62234
800-289-2388

St. Charles, Missouri

First Missouri State Capitol
208-216 South Main Street
St. Charles, MO 63301
314-946-9282
Open April 15 through October, Monday through Saturday, 10 a.m. to 5 p.m.; Sunday, noon to 6 p.m. Open November through mid-April, Monday through Saturday, 10 a.m. to 5 p.m.; Sunday, noon to 5 p.m. Closed on New Year's Day, Easter, Thanksgiving, and Christmas.

Greater St. Charles Convention and Visitors Bureau
230 South Main Street
St. Charles, MO 63301
314-946-7776
800-366-2427
Open Monday through Friday, 8 a.m. to 5 p.m.; Saturday 10 a.m. to 5 p.m.; and Sunday, noon to 5 p.m. Tourist leaflets available.

Shrine of St. Rose Philippine Duchesne
619 North Second Street
St. Charles, MO 63301
314-946-6127
>Open daily 9 a.m. to 4 p.m. Docent tours available; contact shrine for days and times.

KATY Trail

KATY Trail Merchants Group
P.O. Box 1478
Ballwin, MO 63022
314-458-1995

Missouri Department of Natural Resources
P.O. Box 176
Jefferson City, MO 65102
800-334-6946

Appendix C: Great Tastes

St. Louis has countless restaurants offering a variety of cuisines and prices. Have fun exploring the many choices. The restaurants and retail food shops listed below are ones that we loved or that came highly recommended.

Amighetti's

5141 Wilson Avenue
St. Louis, MO 63110
314-776-2855

If the weather is nice, eat your meal on the patio under the shade coverings. Top your Hill visit off with some ice cream.

Balaban's

405 North Euclid
St. Louis, MO 63108
314-361-8085

Among the oldest and most popular of the Central West End restaurants, this moderately priced yet fashionable cafe serves good food in a warm, casual setting. Its huge front windows bring the neighborhood to your table.

Bissinger's French Confections

McPherson Avenue, just east of Euclid Avenue
St. Louis, MO 63108
314-534-2400

This Central West End shop displays its luscious candies in antique cases.

Blueberry Hill Restaurant & Pub

6504 Delmar Boulevard
St. Louis, MO 63130
314-727-0880

No visit to The Loop is complete without a stop at this museum restaurant.

Cunetto House of Pasta
5453 Magnolia Avenue
St. Louis, MO 63139
314-781-1135

Cunetto's on the Hill does not take reservations. So if you do not want to wait, come early in the evening, on a weekday, or for the Monday through Friday lunch. The atmosphere is casual, and the cheese bread is absolutely delicious.

Dickmann's Boulevard Bakery
3139 South Grand
St. Louis, MO 63118
314-773-7585

In this Grand Street shop, rediscover the smells and tastes of an old-fashioned city bakery.

Ted Drewes
6726 Chippewa Street
St. Louis, MO
314-481-2652

You will be able to identify this shop by the long lines that form outside it each evening. Opened in 1929, Drewes serves the best vanilla custard you will find anywhere. This landmark is famous for its "cement," a custard mixed with any number of tasty ingredients and whipped so thick that you can turn it upside down and not lose one delicious drop.

Imo's Pizza
A blend of cheeses gives the pizza from this popular chain a distinct flavor. Voted best pizza in St. Louis by *Riverfront Times*, Imo's has many locations. Check the White Pages for the restaurant nearest you. Enjoy a salad with the house dressing.

Lynch Street Bistro

1031 Lynch Street
St. Louis, MO 63118
314-772-5777

If delicious food graciously served in an inviting atmosphere were not enough, this Soulard bistro also has a collection of paintings by the Beat generation writer William S. Burroughs.

The Majestic

4900 Laclede
St. Louis, MO 63108
314-361-2011

Do not let its plain exterior fool you. This Central West End eatery has it all: neighborhood friendliness, good food, reasonable prices, ample portions, terrific breakfasts, and even patio dining.

Mama Campisi's Restaurant

2132 Edwards Avenue
St. Louis, MO 63110
314-771-1797

Mama Campisi's is one of the few Hill restaurants open on Sundays. The lasagna is especially good, with a nice blend of cheeses and sauce.

Old Spaghetti Factory

727 North First
St. Louis, MO 63102
314-621-0276

Popular and often jam-packed, this restaurant has great atmosphere, good food, and reasonable prices. Children feel right at home in this bustling eatery.

Tony's
410 Market Street
St. Louis, MO 63102
314-231-7007
> *Conde Nast Traveler* rates this downtown Italian restaurant tops in the nation. Reservations highly recommended.

John Viviano and Sons Retail Grocers
5139 Shaw Avenue
St. Louis, MO 63110
314-771-5476
> Even if you do not have a grocery list with you, stop in and feast on the atmosphere.

St. Charles

Café Beignet
515 South Main Street
St. Charles, MO 63301
314-947-3000
> Serves breakfast and lunch in a historic building that dates back to the early 1800s.

Winery of the Little Hills
501 South Main Street
St. Charles, MO 63301
314-946-9339
> Open daily for lunch and dinner. The outdoor dining area includes a large fire pit that warms diners when there is a chill in the air.

Appendix D: Useful Phone Numbers

Please note that the area code for St. Louis is 314.

St. Louis Police:

Emergency, 911

Non-emergency, 444-5555

Fire emergency, 911

Health Care:

Ask-a-Nurse, 645-4500

Barnes-Jewish Hospital, 362-1507

Cardinal Glennon Children's Hospital, 577-5600

Poison Control, 772-5200

St. Anthony Medical Center, 525-1000

Library: 241-2288, main branch

Newspaper:

St. Louis Post-Dispatch, 340-8000

Post Office:

Main office, 436-4453

Missouri State Highway Patrol, 340-4000

Highway conditions, 800-222-6400

Time and Temperature: 321-2522

Weather forecast: 441-8467

Western Union: 800-325-6000

Appendix E: Read All About It

Want to learn more about St. Louis? The following books are but a sample of the many you might enjoy.

Nonfiction

Fifield, Barringer. *Seeing Saint Louis.* St. Louis: Washington University, 1989.

> Engaging black-and-white photos, an eye for the interesting and beautiful, and an informative style makes this book a good choice for anyone interested in the city's history and architecture. Suitable for walkers, the book also includes car tours.

Primm, James Neal. *Lion of the Valley: St. Louis Missouri.* Second edition. Boulder, Colo: Pruett, 1990.

> The author, a professor of history at the University of Missouri-St. Louis, gives readers a comprehensive look at St. Louis. Many black-and-white drawings and photos included.

Fiction

Savan, Glenn. *White Palace.* New York: Bantam, 1987.

> Made into a movie starring Susan Sarandon, *White Palace* is a love story about an advertising copywriter and his passion for a waitress from St. Louis's Dogtown. Filmed in South St. Louis, the movie offers a nice glimpse of the city.

If you like Judy Garland and musicals, by all means watch *Meet Me in St. Louis,* but do not expect to learn anything about St. Louis or the 1904 World's Fair.

Appendix F: Local Walking Clubs

St. Louis-Stuttgart Sister City
6700 Arsenal Street
St. Louis, MO 63139

S.M.T.M. Volkssport Society
1300 New Florissant Road
Florissant, MO 63033-2122

Missouri Woodland Walkers
P.O. Box 1191
St. Charles, MO 63302

Illinois Trekkers Volkssport Club
P.O. Box 25063
Scott AFB, IL 62225-0063

The St. Louis-Stuttgart Sister City walking club is part of the American Volkssport Association, a network of clubs that sponsor non-competitive walking, swimming, and biking events. In St. Charles, walkers will find the S.M.T.M. Volkssport Society and the Missouri Woodland Walkers; and in nearby Illinois, the Illinois Trekkers Volkssport Club, which offers walks in Belleville and Collinsville.

To receive a free information packet that explains volkssporting and the American Volkssport Association, call the AVA at 800-830-WALK and leave your name, address, and phone number.

The AVA office also can provide the local phone contacts for the AVA clubs mentioned above. Many of these clubs sponsor one-day, 5K and 10K (6.2 mile) walking events in the St. Louis area, and the AVA has the dates and locations of these walks.

Index

Page numbers in *italics* refer to photos
Page numbers in **bold** refer to maps